The Chicago Review Press

PHARMACOLOGY MADE EASY
for
NCLEX
RN

Review and Study Guide

Linda Waide, MSN, MEd, RN
and Berta Roland, MSN, RN

Library of Congress Cataloging-in Publication Data is available from the Library of Congress.

This book has been carefully prepared to reflect current standards of nursing practice. As new information becomes available, policies, procedures, drugs, and treatments will change. In determining a plan of care, the practitioner is advised to consult with his or her institution's policies and procedures and with the hospital formulary. The authors and publisher cannot accept any responsibility for errors or omissions or for any consequences resulting from the application of the information in this book, and make no warranty, expressed or implied, with respect to its content. Further, the authors and publisher disclaim all responsibility for any liability, loss, injury, or damage incurred as a direct or indirect consequence of its content.

Published by Chicago Review Press, Incorporated
814 North Franklin Street
Chicago, Illinois 60610

ISBN 1-55652-391-2
Printed in the United States of America

The drug dosages and treatments presented here are compatible with accepted standards at the time of publication. Since pharmacology is a rapidly changing science, the reader is advised to carefully consult the instructional and informational material in the package insert of each medication or therapeutic agent before administration. This advice is especially important when using, administering, or recommending new or infrequently used drugs. The authors and publisher disclaim all responsibility for any liability, loss, injury, or damage incurred as a consequence directly or indirectly in the use and application of any of the contents of this review.

Contents

Acknowledgments

We wish to express our appreciation to the consultants and contributors for their efforts and expertise. It has been very rewarding to associate with such capable and pleasant professionals in the creation of this review and study guide. Because of their valuable assistance, *Pharmacology Made Easy for NCLEX-RN* is now available to help graduates prepare for the RN Licensure Examination.

We also wish to thank Noreen Pitts for her tireless and tenacious efforts in preparing and preparing and preparing the many revisions that came across her desk for *Pharmacology Made Easy for NCLEX-RN*. She exemplifies professionalism on a daily basis.

Consultants and Contributors

Joanne Brown, MSN, MPH, RN
Health Education and Health Promotion
University of Alabama at Birmingham

Jane Case, MSN, FNP, RN
Vanderbilt University, Nashville, Tennessee

Amy Chrapliwy, MSc, BSN, RN
Director, Faith Wesleyan Child Care Center
Greensboro, North Carolina

Judith Cooper, MSN, RN
CNS—Maternal-Infant Care
Assistant Professor, Troy State University, Troy, Alabama

Mary Ann Dell, EdD, RN
Associate Professor, Troy State University, Troy, Alabama
Coordinator of MSN program at Phoenix City, Alabama

Phyllis Horton, MSN, RN
President of Stellar Systems, Education Consultant
Eden, North Carolina

Joyce Jenkins, MSN, RN
Assistant Professor, CNS—Pediatrics
Troy State University, Troy, Alabama

Margaret Lyles, MSN, RN
Assistant Professor, Adult Health Coordinator
Troy State University, Troy, Alabama

Preface

Mastering pharmacology can be a time-consuming, difficult, and sometimes overwhelming task for graduate nurses preparing for the NCLEX-RN. *Pharmacology Made Easy for NCLEX-RN Review and Study Guide* was created to provide graduates with a quick and efficient way to assure their success. This one-of-a-kind text furnishes the graduate with the knowledge and confidence needed to excel in the classroom and on the pharmacology portion of the NCLEX-RN.

Pharmacology Made Easy for NCLEX-RN prepares the graduate for success on the NCLEX in three important ways.

First, it increases the graduate's knowledge of pharmacology with 15 carefully written practice tests that include answers and rationales for every question, plus a 100-question practice test on an interactive software computer disk, also with answers and rationales. All questions follow the latest NCLEX-RN test plan and format. The answers and rationales given at the end of each practice test are designed to teach the graduate **why** the correct answer is right and **why** the three distractions are incorrect. All phases of Client Need (Health Promotion/Maintenance, Physiological Integrity, Psychosocial Integrity, and Safe, Effective Care Environment) are identified for every question. Graduates can easily trace their competence and success in all of these areas.

Second, *Pharmacology Made Easy for NCLEX-RN* gives each graduate an opportunity to practice and learn test-taking skills and strategies that are vital for success on the NCLEX-RN CAT (Computerized Adaptive Testing). Practicing how to select correct answers using the Critical Thinking Process can improve test scores. Graduates who possess good test-taking skills and are able to apply knowledge correctly are more likely to experience success on the NCLEX-RN.

Third, this review decreases test-taking anxiety for licensure candidates. Many graduates tell us they study for tests but are too anxious to remember the subject matter being tested. By preparing for the NCLEX-RN with the *Pharmacology Made Easy for NCLEX-RN Review and Study Guide*, graduates can feel confident because they have prepared appropriately.

Introduction

The Purpose of Drugs

Drugs are used to treat medical diseases, disorders, and conditions. They are also administered for diagnosis and prevention of diseases and disorders, and to maintain health. In addition to prescribed drugs, "over-the-counter" (OTC) drugs such as aspirin, Tagamet, and Benadryl; various salves, ointments, and solutions; and home remedies such as soda and salt are also used to treat and relieve symptoms.

For nursing purposes, drugs can be defined as agents prescribed by qualified health professionals for the treatment of disorders. Since the early 1900s, many laws have been passed by the U.S. Congress to make drugs safer for use. Drugs are now regulated by the federal government through the Food and Drug Administration (FDA). Prior to FDA control, a retroactive system was employed to assess drugs already on the market. Today we have two broad groupings of drugs defined by the Food and Drug Administration: "over-the-counter" and "prescription."

Persons administering and receiving drugs should be aware that drugs alone cannot cure. They combine with the body's natural defenses to bring recovery and stabilization. Where some drugs are helpful for some individuals, for others they may not be effective. Each of us has our own unique immune system. Drugs that bring astounding relief to some will invariably bring no relief to others.

Medications are classified according to their therapeutic uses. Those that have multiple therapeutic uses, like aspirin, are classified according to their most common usage. Drugs can be toxic to the body. Persons administering and receiving drugs should understand the full consequences of any drug given for a particular condition. Individuals will respond differently to the type of drug and dosage administered. Drug regimens should be established with a health-care provider.

Drug Names

There are three different names for every drug. The chemical name describes the drug in terms of its chemistry. Aspirin's chemical name, for instance, is acetylsalicylic acid. Nurses and other health-care providers usually do not refer to a drug by its chemical name when they are communicating with a client or with each other, partly because it is generally difficult to pronounce.

A drug also has a generic or nonproprietary name and at least one trade or brand name. Each drug has only one generic name, while it can have several trade names. "Aspirin" is the generic name for acetylsalicylic acid. Aspirin's trade names include Bayer Aspirin, Bayer Buffered Aspirin, and many more. Trade names are protected by trademark registration. Even though the generic name can be longer and more difficult to pronounce than a trade name, nurses and other health-care professionals generally prefer to use a drug's generic name.

Routes of Drug Absorption

Drugs can be absorbed into the body by three major routes: the enteral, the parenteral, and the percutaneous.

Enteral Route

Drugs administered by the oral, rectal, and nasogastric routes go directly into the gastrointestinal tract. This is the enteral (intestinal) route. Drugs given via the enteral route have the slowest and least dependable rate of absorption, resulting in a slower onset of drug action. Drugs such as insulin and gentamicin are destroyed by digestive fluids and must not be administered enterally.

The enteral route should not be used if the client is experiencing vomiting, gastrointestinal suctioning (where there is a possibility of aspiration), or if the client is unconscious. The enteral route should not be used if the drug harms or discolors the teeth.

Enteral-route medications can be administered as:

- Capsules
- Elixirs
- Emulsions
- Lozenges
- Suspensions
- Syrups
- Tablets

Parenteral Route

When drugs are given parenterally, they do not go through the gastrointestinal tract. The onset of action is usually more rapid but the effects are of shorter duration. Drugs are administered parenterally when they must be absorbed rapidly and at a steady, controlled rate. The parenteral route of administration is also used when the client is experiencing nausea and vomiting. Several different parenteral routes may be used.

Intradermal (ID) Route
Intradermal injections are administered just below the epidermis into the dermis. The absorption rate is slow. This is the route of choice for:

- Allergy sensitivity
- Desensitization
- Local anesthetics
- Vaccinations
- Intramuscular (IM) Route

Intramuscular injections are carried out by the use of a needle penetrating the dermis and subcutaneous tissue and entering into the muscle tissue. The drug is deposited into the muscle mass. Absorption is more rapid with IM injections due to greater blood supply to the muscles. Injections should be made into healthy tissue with careful placement of the needle so that damage to nerves and blood vessels is avoided.

Intravenous (IV) Route
The intravenous route places the drug directly into the bloodstream. Intravenous administration is the most rapid of all the parenteral routes. Large volumes of drugs can be administered into the vein, usually with little irritation. Most of the time IV medications are given on an intermittent basis, or the drug can be given continuously through an established IV line. The IV route is usually the most comfortable for the client if the drugs are to be given daily for several days.

Subcutaneous (SC) Route
Subcutaneous injections are made into the subcutaneous tissue, the loose connective tissue located between the dermis and the muscle layer. Many drugs cannot be administered by the subcutaneous route because only 2 ml of fluid can be injected into subcutaneous tissue at one time. If circulation is adequate, subcutaneous injections are completely absorbed. Examples of drugs commonly injected subcutaneously are:

- Heparin
- Insulin

Sometimes the terms intralesional (into a lesion), intra-arterial (into an artery), intracardiac (into the heart), intra-articular (into a joint), or intrathecal (within the spinal cord) are used.

Percutaneous Route

Percutaneous administration refers to the application of medication to the skin or mucus membranes. Absorption can be influenced by the drug's concentration, the length of contact with the skin, affected areas, size of affected areas, thickness of the skin, tissue hydration, and how much the skin has been disrupted. The primary advantage of percutaneous administration is localization that reduces systemic side effects. Medications given via the percutaneous route may be difficult to apply, messy, and time-consuming due to the short duration of their action. These drugs require frequent application. Percutaneous administration can be made via:

- Creams
- Inhalants
- Instillations
- Lotions
- Patches
- Powders

Practice Test 1

Anti-Infective Agents

OVERVIEW

Anti-infectives are natural or synthetic compounds that treat, inhibit, and prevent various kinds of infections.

Anti-infectives include:

- **Amebicides and antiprotozoals**
- **Aminoglycosides**
- **Anthelmintics**
- **Antifungals**
- **Antimalarials**
- **Antituberculars and antileprotics**
- **Antivirals**
- **Cephalosporins**
- **Macrolides**
- **Penicillins**
- **Quinolones**
- **Sulfonamides**
- **Tetracyclines**

AMEBICIDES AND ANTIPROTOZOALS

AMEBICIDES are substances that kill amebas. A person infected with amebas is said to have amebiasis. Amebiasis is caused by the parasite Entamoeba histolytica.

There are two types of amebiasis: intestinal and extraintestinal. The extraintestinal type, such as that found in the liver, is more difficult to treat.

Conditions treated with amebicides include:

- Amebic dysentery
- Amebic hepatitis

ANTIPROTOZOALS are substances that kill protozoa. Protozoa are single-celled parasitic organisms. Protozoal infections are typically spread by the fecal-oral route where food or water is contaminated with cysts or spores. Infections may also occur through the bite of a mosquito or other insect that has previously bitten an infected person.

Conditions treated with antiprotozoals include:

- Sleeping sickness (Trypanosoma gambiense)
- Vaginal infections (Trichomonas vaginalis)

AMINOGLYCOSIDES

Aminoglycosides are chemical compounds found in some anti-infectives. Some of these compounds are derived from microorganisms while others are produced synthetically. Aminoglycosides are effective in treating bacterial infections (especially those caused by gram-negative microorganisms).

Conditions treated with aminoglycosides include:

- Urinary tract infections (UTIs)
- Wound infections
- Septicemia

Aminoglycosides may also be used to decrease the number of normal intestinal flora prior to gastrointestinal surgery.

ANTHELMINTICS

Anthelmintics are substances used to treat people who are infected with worms (helminths). The most common infections are associated with hookworms, pinworms, roundworms, tapeworms, and whipworms.

To determine the treatment of choice, the type of worm must be identified. This is done by examination of the stool for the ova (eggs) or the worm itself.

Conditions treated with anthelmintics include:

- Pinworm infection (Enterobius vermicularis)
- Tapeworm infection (Echinococcus granulosus)

ANTIFUNGALS

Antifungal agents hinder or slow the multiplication of fungi (fungistatics) or destroy the fungi (fungicides). Fungal infections are referred to as myotic infections. These infections may be superficial or systemic. Superficial infections would include conditions of the skin and nails. Systemic infections are those occurring inside the body.

Fungi include yeast and molds and are found in the air, soil, and water. Only a few will cause disease.

Conditions treated with antifungals include:

- Histoplasmosis (disease of the lungs)
- Ringworm (skin infection)
- Candidiasis (local and systemic infection)
- Athlete's foot (skin infection)
- Thrush (mouth and throat infection)

ANTIMALARIALS

An antimalarial is prescribed to treat persons with malaria. Malaria is transmitted to humans through the bite of an anopheles mosquito infected with one of the four protozoa that cause malaria (Plasmodium falciparum, Plasmodium malariae, Plasmodium ovale, Plasmodium vivax).

Antimalarial substances are used to suppress (prevent) malaria or to manage (treat) an acute attack of malaria.

Conditions treated with antimalarials include:

- Acute malarial attacks
- Malaria (as suppressive prophylaxis)

ANTITUBERCULARS AND ANTILEPROTICS

ANTITUBERCULARS are used to treat people who have tuberculosis. Tuberculosis is caused by the Mycobacterium tuberculosis bacillus. Treatment of tuberculosis usually includes the administration of two or more antitubercular medications.

Persons receiving two or more medications from the same drug classification are doing so for the drugs' synergistic action (together, the drugs produce a therapeutic effect that neither drug could produce alone).

Conditions treated with antituberculars include:

- Pulmonary tuberculosis (infection of the lung)
- Miliary tuberculosis (tuberculosis infection that spreads throughout the body)
- Open tuberculosis (tuberculosis infection where the bacilli are present in the secretions that leave the body)

ANTILEPROTICS are administered to treat people who have leprosy (Hansen's disease). Leprosy is caused by the microorganism Mycobacterium leprae.

The two main types of leprosy are lepromatous and tuberculoid. Lepromatous leprosy is characterized by skin lesions and involvement of peripheral nerves. Tuberculoid leprosy involves asymmetrical nerve and skin lesions with anesthesia of the skin.

Conditions treated with antileprotics include:

- Lepromatous leprosy
- Tuberculoid leprosy

ANTIVIRALS

Antivirals treat conditions caused by viruses. Antiviral medications are effective only in a small number of very specific infections caused by viruses.

Conditions treated with antivirals include:

- Influenza A (treatment/prevention)
- Retinitis
- Herpes simplex
- Acquired immunodeficiency syndrome (AIDS)

CEPHALOSPORINS

Cephalosporins are structurally related to penicillins. They are used to treat infections in which the microorganisms are susceptible. Cephalosporins may also be used when people are found to be allergic to penicillins.

Cephalosporins are separated into first-, second-, and third-generation medications. Generally speaking, the first-generation cephalosporins are more effective in treating gram-positive microorganisms such as streptococci and some strains of staphylococci. The second-generation cephalosporins are effective against the organisms of the first generation and also against Haemophilus influenzae. The third-generation cephalosporins are more effective in treating gram-negative organisms.

Conditions treated with cephalosporins include:

- Urinary tract infections (UTIs)
- Abdominal infections
- Septicemia
- Meningitis
- Osteomyelitis

MACROLIDES

Macrolides are any of a group of antibacterial anti-infectives produced by certain species of streptomyces.

Conditions treated with macrolides include:

- Streptococcus pneumonia
- S. pyogens pharyngitis/tonsillitis
- Haemophilus influenzae

PENICILLINS

Penicillins have antibacterial properties that are used to treat infections that are susceptible to them. It is necessary to perform culture and sensitivity tests to see which penicillin will be most effective in treating a particular infection.

Penicillins may treat infection by actually killing bacteria (bactericidal) or slowing down the multiplication/reproduction of bacteria (bacteriostatic). Occasionally penicillins are used as a prophylaxis (to prevent infection).

Conditions treated with penicillins include:

- Pneumonia
- Otitis media
- Urinary tract infections (UTIs)
- Rheumatic fever
- Syphilis
- Meningitis
- Gonorrhea

QUINOLONES

Quinolones are broad-spectrum anti-infectives that are absorbed rapidly from the gastrointestinal tract. Quinolones have a low incidence of adverse reactions. A subcategory of quinolones is the fluoroquinolones.

Conditions treated with quinolones include:

- Urinary tract infections (UTIs)
- Gonorrhea
- Lower respiratory tract infections
- Skin infections
- Conjunctivitis

SULFONAMIDES

Sulfonamides are not true anti-infectives because they are not synthesized by microorganisms. They are, however, very effective antibacterial agents.

Conditions treated with sulfonamides include:

- Urinary tract infections (UTIs)
- Otitis media
- Streptococcal infection associated with rheumatic fever (as a prophylaxis)

TETRACYCLINES

Tetracyclines are effective against both gram-negative and gram-positive bacteria. Tetracyclines may be used in cases of penicillin allergy. Tetracyclines are very effective when treating conditions caused by rickettsial and mycoplasmic organisms.

Conditions treated with tetracyclines include:

- Urinary tract infections (UTIs)
- Upper respiratory tract infections
- Pneumonia
- Meningitis
- Venereal diseases

Practice Test 1

Questions

1 - 1

A pediatric client who experienced chickenpox recently has been diagnosed with erysipelas or "St. Anthony's fire." For which of the following do you anticipate a prescription?

1. diphenhydramine (Benadryl)
2. famciclovir (Famvir)
3. penicillin G procaine (Crysticillin)
4. folic acid (vitamin B₉)

1 - 2

Your client has been diagnosed with schistosomiasis (a parasitic disease). Oxamniquine (Vansil) has been prescribed. A part of the client's history that would be very important to know would be:

1. lactose intolerance.
2. febrile reaction to antibiotics.
3. peptic ulcer disease.
4. seizure disorder.

1 - 3

A family arrives at your clinic. Two of the 5 children are diagnosed with pinworms. Pyrantel pamoate (Pin-X) has been prescribed. Regarding the administration of this medication, you know that:

1. it is contraindicated in children under 3 years old.
2. it is taken daily for 7 consecutive days.
3. only the 2 affected children will need to take the medication.
4. this drug may cause seizures.

1 - 4

Your client has just had a colon resection and the following medication was prescribed: metronidazole (Flagyl) 5 gm intravenously every 6 hours. You will know to:

1. hold this medication and notify the physician.
2. give the medication immediately.
3. give the medication intramuscularly.
4. begin the medication on the second post-operative day.

1 - 5

A client with chronic obstructive pulmonary disease (COPD) is being treated with a Beclovent inhaler, theophylline by mouth, and steroids daily. Thiabendazole (Mintezol) is to be administered for the treatment of roundworms. You will monitor the client for:

1. digoxin toxicity.
2. theophylline toxicity.
3. constipation.
4. weight gain.

1 - 6

The urine culture of a client is positive for gram-negative bacilli. A gentamicin (Garamycin) intravenous infusion is prescribed. To assess for early side effects of gentamicin, the nurse will closely monitor the client for:

1. an elevated serum level of blood urea nitrogen (BUN) and creatinine.
2. a decrease in urine output.
3. an elevated blood pressure.
4. nausea and vomiting.

1 - 7

The physician has written a prescription for cefoxitin (Mefoxin) 1 gm intravenously every 4 hours. You know this medication is frequently prescribed for:

1. urinary tract infections.
2. elevated body temperature.
3. diarrhea.
4. dysuria.

1 - 8

A client with a fungal skin infection has been taking amphotericin B (Fungizone) and has recently begun taking flucytosine (Ancobon). Regarding the concurrent use of these medications, you know that:

1. they should not be taken concurrently.
2. the amphotericin B dosage must be increased if taken concurrently with flucytosine.
3. the risk of toxic effects increases with concurrent use of these medications.
4. there is no synergistic effect with these medications.

1 - 9

After notifying the physician of green purulent drainage from the pin site of a client's skeletal traction, you anticipate receiving a prescription for:

1. atropine (Atropair).
2. ceftriaxone (Rocephin).
3. bumetanide (Bumex).
4. alteplase (Activase).

1 - 1 0

Your client is to be given pentamidine isethionate (Pentam) for pneumocystis carinii pneumonia. Regarding the administration of this medication, you know:

1. it is contraindicated for those who are positive for the human immunodeficiency virus.
2. it may only be given by mouth.
3. it may not be given intramuscularly.
4. it may be given as an inhalant.

1 - 1 1

Your client has developed a severe systemic fungal infection. Amphotericin B (Fungizone) intravenous has been prescribed. You know this medication:

1. may only be given by mouth.
2. is compatible with most medications given intravenously.
3. is given over 20 to 30 minutes intravenously.
4. is potentially nephrotoxic.

1 - 1 2

A client with diabetes has been diagnosed with a vaginal infection for which she is to use nystatin vaginal suppositories. Included in your teaching plan will be instructions to:

1. discontinue the use of vaginal medications during menstruation.
2. discontinue insulin regimen while on nystatin therapy.
3. use vaginal suppositories as a one-time-only dose.
4. notify the physician of any vaginal swelling or irritation.

1 - 1 3

Your 5-year-old client has been diagnosed with roundworms and is to be given mebendazole (Vermox). You know the administration of this drug:

1. is contraindicated in persons under 10 years of age.
2. is contraindicated in persons with benzodiazepine allergy.
3. is to be given as a one-time dose.
4. should be given to the entire family.

1 - 1 4

Your client has cirrhosis of the liver and is receiving neomycin (Mycifradin). The nurse knows the purpose of this medication is to:

1. prevent gastrointestinal bleeding.
2. decrease the formation of ammonia.
3. acidify the stool in the bowel.
4. reduce fluid volume while sparing potassium.

1 - 1 5

Which of the following medications might be prescribed for a client with osteomyelitis?

1. a cephalosporin antibiotic such as cefotaxime
2. an antifungal agent such as miconazole
3. an antiviral agent such as acyclovir
4. an antiarrhythmic such as verapamil

1 - 1 6

A client diagnosed with cystitis would likely be prescribed medication from which drug category?

1. diuretics
2. antiarrhythmics
3. anti-infectives
4. antineoplastics

1 - 1 7

You will administer an oral suspension of ampicillin, 78 mg/kg qid, to a child who weighs 31 pounds. You know to administer:

1. 10.5 mg.
2. 26 mg.
3. 262.5 mg.
4. 1050 mg.

1 - 1 8

Your client has sustained a grade III open fracture. You will anticipate a prescription for an:

1. antiarrhythmic.
2. anticholinergic.
3. anti-infective.
4. antimetabolite.

1 - 1 9

A client with intestinal parasites is to be discharged with a prescription for iodoquinol (Yodoxin). A contraindication to this therapy would be a drug allergy to:

1. quinine.
2. codeine.
3. penicillin.
4. iodine.

1 - 2 0

Your client is 3 days postoperative following intestinal surgery and has been receiving metronidazole (Flagyl) intravenously. Regarding the administration of this medication, you know that:

1. double-gloving is recommended during the administration of metronidazole.
2. metronidazole is safe to give repeatedly without concern for superinfections.
3. the oral form of metronidazole is to be taken on an empty stomach.
4. metronidazole use may cause the urine to be discolored.

1 - 2 1

A client who uses birth control pills for contraception is to take a course of penicillin antibiotics to treat bronchitis. What will you advise the client to do?

1. Increase the birth control pill dosage.
2. Stop taking the birth control pills while taking the antibiotic.
3. Stop taking the antibiotic as soon as symptoms disappear.
4. Use an additional birth control method while taking antibiotics.

1 - 2 2

Which of the following medications places a client at risk for developing aplastic anemia?

1. chloramphenicol (Chloromycetin)
2. nystatin (Mycostatin)
3. paroxetine (Paxil)
4. mumps virus vaccine

1 - 2 3

A client has been placed on oral tetracycline 250 mg every 6 hours for leg ulcers. For optimum effects, tetracycline should be given:

1. 1 hour before meals.
2. with milk.
3. in orange juice.
4. with meals.

1 - 2 4

Your client has vaginitis caused by the microorganism Trichomonas vaginalis. Four 500-mg tablets of metronidazole (Flagyl) have been prescribed. Which of the following instructions will you give the client regarding the administration of this medication?

1. "Take all 4 tablets at once."
2. "Take 1 tablet a day for 4 days."
3. "You should only consume alcohol in moderation while taking this medicine."
4. "This medication is for symptomatic relief only. There is no cure for this infection."

1 - 2 5

Your client contracted giardiasis after drinking water from a stream contaminated with the protozoan Giardia lamblia. To treat this condition, you will administer metronidazole 750 mg po, tid for 5 to 10 days. You will teach the client the following information about this medication:

1. The drug should be taken on an empty stomach.
2. Sexual partners should be treated simultaneously.
3. The drug may cause the urine to turn light green in color.
4. The drug may cause a sour taste in the mouth.

1 - 2 6

A client with chronic obstructive pulmonary disease (COPD) was admitted with an acute respiratory infection. A course of antibiotic therapy has been completed. The client continues to have a low-grade fever and the tongue is coated. Fluconazole (Diflucan) 100 mg intravenously every 12 hours has been prescribed. This drug is given to treat:

1. gram-negative infections.
2. fungal infections.
3. drug sensitivity.
4. bronchoconstriction.

1 - 2 7

A client is receiving isoniazid (INH) to treat pulmonary tuberculosis. You will monitor the client for which one of the following reactions?

1. hepatitis
2. arthralgia
3. nephrotoxicity
4. ototoxicity

1 - 2 8

Your client is pregnant and is experiencing a chlamydial infection. The drug of choice is:

1. acyclovir (Zovirax).
2. penicillin (Bicillin).
3. erythromycin (Erythrocin).
4. clotrimazole (Lotrimin).

1 - 2 9

Your client received gentamicin sulfate (Garamycin) 3 mg/kg q 8 hours to treat a life-threatening infection. Following the administration of this drug, the client complained of nausea and vomiting. Fluid balance indicates: Blood urea nitrogen 46 mg/dl, creatinine 2.6 mg/l, sodium 148 mEq/l, potassium 4.8 mEq/l. You know these laboratory results suggest:

1. fluid deficit.
2. hypokalemia.
3. fluid overload.
4. acute renal failure.

1 - 3 0

The mother of 4 children ages 3 to 8 years has roundworms. Mebendazole (Vermox) is to be administered. You will teach the mother that:

1. the drug cannot be administered to children.
2. enemas must be given twice daily following the administration of this drug.
3. it is not advisable for an infected person to prepare meals for the family.
4. this drug will need to be taken prophylactically for up to 1 year.

Practice Test 1

Answers, Rationales, and Explanations

1 - 1

③ You will anticipate a prescription for penicillin G procaine (Crysticillin). "St. Anthony's Fire" presents as a very red rash (therefore the name). It is due to a bacterial infection that enters the skin. If abrasions or lesions break the skin, such as the macular papular vesicles associated with chickenpox, the antibiotic penicillin G procaine is the treatment of choice.

1. Diphenhydramine (Benadryl) is administered for allergic reactions and has no significant impact on bacterial infections.
2. Famciclovir (Famvir) is administered for viral infections and has no impact on bacterial infections.
4. Folic acid (vitamin B_9) is a water-soluble vitamin used in the treatment of anemia and has no impact on bacterial infections.

Pregnancy Category: B
Client Need: Physiological Integrity

1 - 2

④ It would be important to know if clients receiving oxamniquine (Vansil) have a history of seizures, since seizures have occurred after administration of this drug. Oxamniquine (Vansil) is an anthelmintic (kills parasitic worms).

1. Lactose intolerance would have no bearing on oxamniquine (Vansil) therapy.
2. Oxamniquine (Vansil) is an anthelmintic, not an antibiotic.
3. Although irritating to the stomach, oxamniquine (Vansil) is not likely to increase the risk of developing peptic ulcers.

Pregnancy Category: C
Client Need: Safe, Effective Care Environment

1 - 3

④ Pyrantel pamoate (Pin-X) may cause seizures. Other central nervous system symptoms include impaired mental alertness, numbness, dizziness, and headache.

1. Pyrantel pamoate (Pin-X) may be given to children as young as 2 years old.
2. For the treatment of pinworms, pyrantel pamoate (Pin-X) is taken as a single dose (11 mg/kg) po. The maximum dosage should not exceed 1 gram.
3. All family members will need treatment due to the high risk of infestation.

Pregnancy Category: B
Client Need: Health Promotion/Maintenance

1 - 4

(1) **The anti-infective metronidazole (Flagyl) should be held and the physician should be notified. A 5-gm intravenous administration of metronidazole (Flagyl) every 6 hours is atypical. The average dose is 500 mg intravenously every 6 to 12 hours. Dosages above 4 grams per day are not recommended.**

2. Five grams every 6 hours exceeds the recommended dosage, and therefore should not be given.

3. Five grams every 6 hours is excessive. Flagyl can only be given by mouth, intravenously, vaginally, and topically, not intramuscularly.

4. Five grams every 6 hours is excessive. Also, to prevent infection, the medication should be given immediately following surgery, not on the second postoperative day.

Pregnancy Category: B
Client Need: Health Promotion/Maintenance

1 - 5

(2) **You will monitor the client for theophylline toxicity. Thiabendazole (Mintezol) may alter theophylline metabolism and increase the risk for toxic accumulation of theophylline. Thiabendazole (Mintezol) inhibits the helminth-specific enzyme fumarate reductase and is used to treat roundworms.**

1. There is no indication that the client is taking digoxin.

3. Thiabendazole (Mintezol) tends to cause diarrhea rather than constipation.

4. There is no indication that thiabendazole (Mintezol) causes weight gain.

Pregnancy Category: C
Client Need: Safe, Effective Care Environment

1 - 6

(1) **The nurse will monitor the client for elevated serum levels of blood urea nitrogen (BUN) and creatinine. Gentamicin is an anti-infective administered for the treatment of gram-negative bacillary infections. Adverse reactions include nephrotoxicity (damage to kidney cells). Early signs of nephrotoxicity can be detected by elevated serum blood urea nitrogen and creatinine levels.**

2, 3, and 4. Decrease in urine output, elevated blood pressure, and nausea and vomiting are later signs of impaired renal function.

Pregnancy Category: C
Client Need: Health Promotion/Maintenance

1 - 7

(1) **Cefoxitin (Mefoxin) is an antibiotic frequently prescribed for the treatment of urinary tract infections caused by gram-positive cocci.**

2. Cefoxitin is not an antipyretic and has no direct effect on body temperature. However, controlling infection may lower body temperature.

3. Cefoxitin is not given to manage diarrhea; one of the side effects of cefoxitin is diarrhea.

4. Cefoxitin is an antibiotic and has no direct effect on dysuria (painful or difficult voiding). Dysuria decreases with the control of infection.

Pregnancy Category: B

Client Need: Physiological Integrity

1 - 8

(3) **The risk of toxic effects increases with concurrent use of amphotericin B (Fungizone) and flucytosine (Ancobon). Amphotericin B and flucytosine have a synergistic effect (the total effects of the two drugs are greater than the sum of the separate effects of the two drugs), and therefore the hepatic, renal, and hematologic toxic effects may be increased.**

1. Amphotericin B and flucytosine may be used concurrently.

2. Amphotericin B and flucytosine have a synergistic effect and both manage fungal infections. However, the Amphotericin B should not be increased.

4. Amphotericin B and flucytosine do potentiate each other in the management of fungal infections.

Pregnancy Category: flucytosine, C; amphotericin B, B

Client Need: Physiological Integrity

1 - 9

(2) **Ceftriaxone (Rocephin) may be prescribed since it is an anti-infective agent (third-generation cephalosporin). The pin site of a skeletal traction is a port of entry for microorganisms and must be assessed carefully for any sign of infection, such as green purulent drainage.**

1. Atropine (Atropair) is an anticholinergic, antiarrhythmic, and ophthalmic. This medication does not treat or prevent infection.

3. Bumetanide (Bumex) is a loop diuretic and does not treat or prevent infection.

4. Alteplase (Activase) is a tissue plasminogen activator that lyses thrombi such as those found in the coronary arteries during an acute myocardial infarction. This medication does not treat or prevent infection.

Pregnancy Category: B

Client Need: Physiological Integrity

1 - 1 0

④ **Pentamidine isethionate (Pentam) may be given as an inhalant. It is an anti-infective (antiprotozoal). Giving this medication as an inhalant is the usual route of administration for the prevention and treatment of pneumocystis carinii pneumonia, an opportunistic disease of clients with human immunodeficiency virus—HIV/acquired immune deficiency syndrome—AIDS.**

1. Pentamidine isethionate (Pentam) is prescribed for clients who are positive for the human immunodeficiency virus (HIV). It is given to prevent and treat pneumocystis carinii pneumonia.

2 and 3. Pentamidine isethionate (Pentam) may be given by mouth, intravenously, intramuscularly, or as an inhalant.

Pregnancy Category: C
Client Need: Health Promotion/Maintenance

1 - 1 1

④ **Amphotericin B is an antifungal agent that is nephrotoxic (damages kidney cells.) Weekly renal function studies are recommended to monitor blood urea nitrogen (BUN) and creatinine.**

1. Presently in the United States the oral form is unavailable. The intravenous route is most commonly used. There is also a topical form of this medicine.

2. Amphotericin B is notorious for incompatibility with most other medications in solution.

3. Amphotericin B should be given over a 6-hour period due to serious cardiovascular side effects.

Pregnancy Category: B
Client Need: Physiological Integrity

1 - 1 2

④ **Any vaginal swelling or irritation may be a reaction to the nystatin vaginal suppositories and should be reported. Nystatin vaginal suppositories are antifungal agents.**

1. Nystatin vaginal suppositories may be continued throughout menstruation.

2. The insulin regimen should not be interrupted unless the client is being treated for fluctuations in serum glucose levels.

3. Nystatin vaginal suppositories are usually prescribed for 10 to 14 days.

Pregnancy Category: A
Client Need: Health Promotion/Maintenance

1 - 1 3

④ **Due to the high incidence of familial infestation, it is recommended that the entire family be treated for roundworms. This medication is also used to treat whipworms, pinworms, and hookworms.**

1. Mebendazole (Vermox) may be given to persons over 2 years of age.
2. There is no indication that a person with a benzodiazepine (Librium and Valium) allergy will be allergic to mebendazole (Vermox).
3. For treatment of roundworms, whipworms, and hookworms, 100 mg of mebendazole (Vermox) is given by mouth twice daily for 3 days. For the treatment of pinworms, 100 mg by mouth is given as a one-time dosage.

Pregnancy Category: C
Client Need: Physiological Integrity

1 - 1 4

② **Neomycin (Mycifradin) is an anti-infective that decreases the formation of ammonia. A major concern for clients with cirrhosis of the liver is the complication of hepatic encephalopathy (hepatic coma) caused by excess ammonia in the blood. Neomycin decreases the bacterial flora in the gastrointestinal tract and thus decreases the formation of ammonia.**

1. Inderal-LA, not neomycin (Mycifradin), is an antihypertensive that is commonly prescribed for clients with cirrhosis of the liver to lower blood pressure and prevent gastrointestinal bleeding.
3. Lactulose, not neomycin (Mycifradin), is a laxative (hyperosmotic) that acidifies the feces in the bowel and traps ammonia, causing it to be eliminated in the feces.
4. Spironolactone, not neomycin (Mycifradin), is an example of a potassium-sparing diuretic that reduces fluid volume. It has no impact on ammonia in the blood.

Pregnancy Category: D
Client Need: Physiological Integrity

1 - 1 5

① **A cephalosporin antibiotic such as cefotaxime is an effective treatment for osteomyelitis. Osteomyelitis (infection in the bone) is a potentially morbid disorder that may spread to surrounding tissue. Osteomyelitis is commonly caused by the microorganism staphylococcus aureus, which is susceptible to treatment with cephalosporin or penicillin antibiotics.**

2. Antifungal agents such as miconazole have no impact on staphylococcus aureus.
3. Antiviral agents such as acyclovir have no impact on staphylococcus aureus.
4. Antiarrhythmics such as verapamil have no impact on staphylococcus aureus.

Pregnancy Category: B
Client Need: Physiological Integrity

1 - 1 6

③ **Anti-infective therapy with antibiotics such as sulfonamides is typically prescribed for clients with cystitis (inflammation of the urinary bladder). Cystitis is often caused by the microorganism E. coli, which is normally found in the bowel.**

1. Diuretics are indicated only if excess fluid needs to be excreted.
2. Antiarrhythmics are prescribed if a cardiac rhythm disturbance is evidenced.
4. Antineoplastic medications are prescribed to treat cancer.

Pregnancy Category: Varies with specific drug
Client Need: Physiological Integrity

1 - 1 7

④ **A child who weighs 31 pounds (14 kg) should receive 1050 mg of the ampicillin qid (75 mg x 14 kg = 1050 mg).**

1, 2, and 3. 10.5 mg, 26 mg, and 262.5 mg are incorrect amounts.

Pregnancy Category: C
Client Need: Physiological Integrity

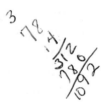

1 - 1 8

③ **A prescription for an anti-infective is anticipated. A grade III open fracture is an extensive injury with soft tissue damage caused by the protrusion of bone fragments. Because of the exposure of bone and tissue, the risk of infection is great and anti-infectives would be indicated to avoid this complication.**

1. Antiarrhythmics are prescribed to treat cardiac arrhythmias and have no impact on infection.
2. Anticholinergics affect the nervous system and have no impact on infection.
4. Antimetabolites adversely affect cell growth and have no impact on infection.

Pregnancy Category: Varies with specific drug
Client Need: Physiological Integrity

1 - 1 9

④ **Iodoquinol (Yodoxin) is an iodine derivative. Persons allergic to iodine would be allergic to iodoquinol.**

1, 2, and 3. There is no indication that allergies to quinine, codeine, or penicillin would affect iodoquinol use.

Pregnancy Category: C
Client Need: Health Promotion/Maintenance

1 - 2 0

④   **The metabolites (substances produced during metabolism) of metronidazole may cause urine to turn dark.**

1.   There is no indication that double-gloving is necessary when administering metronidazole. However, when preparing some intravenous antineoplastic medications such as methotrexate, the nurse should glove, gown, and mask since direct contact with cytotoxic drugs may cause irritation of skin, eyes, and mucous membranes.

2.   Clients should be informed that superinfections may occur. They should observe for furry overgrowth on tongue, vaginal itching, and loose stools.

3.   The oral form of this medication should be given with food to minimize gastric irritation.

Pregnancy Category: B
Client Need: Physiological Integrity

1 - 2 1

④   **An additional birth control method should be used during penicillin therapy. Some antibiotics have been found to affect gastrointestinal flora and thereby interfere with the absorption and metabolism of birth control pills.**

1 and 2. An alternative birth control method should be implemented.

3.   Antibiotic therapy should not be stopped until the course is complete.

Pregnancy Category: Varies with specific drug
Client Need: Physiological Integrity

1 - 2 2

①   **Clients receiving chloramphenicol (Chloromycetin) are at risk for developing aplastic anemia. Aplastic anemia is an anemia resulting from bone marrow suppression. Chloramphenicol is a potent anti-infective whose impact on protein synthesis may also affect bone marrow. Clients should be assessed daily for signs of bone marrow depression such as sore throat, petechiae, bleeding, and bruising.**

2, 3, and 4. Neither nystatin (Mycostatin), paroxetine (Paxil), or mumps virus vaccine is known to cause bone marrow suppression.

Pregnancy Category: C
Client Need: Health Promotion/Maintenance

1 - 2 3

1. For optimum effect, it is recommended that tetracycline be given 1 hour before meals. Tetracycline should be given on an empty stomach because food, milk, and milk products can reduce absorption by 50%.

2. Dairy products are known to bind tetracycline and prevent absorption; therefore, tetracycline should not be given with milk.

3 and 4. Tetracycline should be given on an empty stomach, not in orange juice or with meals.

Pregnancy Category: D

Client Need: Physiological Integrity

1 - 2 4

1. You will teach the client that all four 500-mg tablets of metronidazole (Flagyl) should be taken at once. The microorganism Trichomonas vaginalis is a resilient flagellum that can be successfully treated with metronidazole. It is important that 2 grams of the medication be taken at one time in order for the serum levels of the medication to be adequate to kill the microorganisms.

2. All four 500-mg tablets of metronidazole (Flagyl) should be taken at once, not one once a day for 4 days.

3. Alcohol is contraindicated during the course of metronidazole (Flagyl) administration, due to the likelihood of nausea and vomiting.

4. Vaginitis caused by the organism Trichomonas vaginalis is a treatable sexually transmitted disease.

Pregnancy Category: B

Client Need: Physiological Integrity

1 - 2 5

2. You will teach your client that sexual partners should be treated simultaneously to avoid reinfection. Giardiasis is an infection of the small bowel caused by the protozoan Giardia lamblia. The contaminated feces of infected clients can pass the condition to others.

1. Metronidazole (Flagyl) should be taken with meals to minimize gastrointestinal upset.

3. The urine of clients taking metronidazole (Flagyl) may turn dark or a red-brown color.

4. A metallic taste in the mouth may occur when taking metronidazole (Flagyl).

Pregnancy Category: B

Client Need: Physiological Integrity

1 - 2 6

② **Fluconazole (Diflucan) is given to treat fungal infections. Long-term antibiotic therapy may affect the normal bacterial flora of the host (client) as well as the offending microorganisms. As a result, persons on long-term antibiotic therapy are more prone to fungal infections.**

1. Upper respiratory and urinary tract infections caused by gram-negative bacilli such as E. coli and klebsiella are not treated with antifungal medications.

3. Drug sensitivity is often manifested by a skin rash and treated by discontinuing the drug responsible.

4. Fluconazole (Diflucan) is an antifungal, not a bronchodilator, and has no impact on bronchoconstriction.

Pregnancy Category: C

Client Need: Physiological Integrity

1 - 2 7

① **Adverse reactions associated with the administration of isoniazid (INH) include hepatitis and peripheral neuropathy. Hepatitis may be severe and occasionally fatal in the elderly.**

2. Arthralgia (joint pain) is not associated with the administration of isoniazid. However, it is associated with rifampin, which is a commonly administered antitubercular drug.

3. Nephrotoxicity is not associated with the administration of isoniazid. However, it is associated with streptomycin, which is commonly administered to treat tuberculosis.

4. Ototoxicity is not associated with the administration of isoniazid. However, it is associated with streptomycin, which is commonly administered to treat tuberculosis.

Pregnancy Category: C

Client Need: Physiological Integrity

1 - 2 8

③ **The drug of choice for treating a pregnant woman with a chlamydial infection is erythromycin (Erythrocin). The ophthalmic form of erythromycin (erythromycin 0.5 ophthalmic ointment) is given to all newborns as a prophylaxis for ophthalmia neonatorum.**

1. Acyclovir (Zovirax) is used to treat herpes simplex and h. zoster infections.

2. Penicillin (Bicillin) may be given to treat congenital syphilis.

4. Clotrimazole (Lotrimin) is useful in treating candida.

Pregnancy Category: B

Client Need: Physiological Integrity

1 - 2 9

④ **This client is in renal failure. A blood urea nitrogen (BUN) of 46 mg/dl and a creatinine of 2.6 mg/l indicate renal failure. Normal BUN levels are 5 to 20 mg/dl. Normal creatinine levels are 0.7 to 1.5 mg/dl.**

1. With fluid deficit, there would be an increase in the BUN levels. However, creatinine is less likely to be affected.

2. Normal potassium levels are 3.5 to 5.5 mEq/l. Therefore, a potassium level of 4.8 mEq/l is within normal limits and does not indicate hypokalemia.

3. Normal sodium levels are 135 to 148 mEq/l. The sodium level of 148 mEq/l and the BUN of 46 mg/dl do not suggest fluid overload.

Pregnancy Category: D

Client Need: Physiological Integrity

1 - 3 0

③ **You will teach the mother (client) that it is not advisable for her to prepare food because of the likelihood of infecting those who will be eating the food. The client should be taught about personal hygiene, good hand-washing technique, and changing undergarments and bedclothes daily. The entire family should be treated concurrently.**

1. Mebendazole (Vermox) may be administered to adults and children over 2 years old.

2. Neither enemas nor laxatives are recommended following the administration of Vermox. The drug may cause nausea, vomiting, diarrhea, and abdominal cramps.

4. To treat roundworms, Mebendazole (Vermox) is administered as a 100-mg po tablet. It may be repeated if infection lasts 2 to 3 weeks thereafter.

Pregnancy Category: C

Client Need: Health Promotion/Maintenance

Practice Test 2

Antineoplastic Agents

OVERVIEW

Antineoplastics are administered to destroy or prevent the development, growth, and proliferation of malignant cells. People receiving antineoplastic agents are said to be receiving chemotherapy.

Antineoplastics include:

- **Alkylating agents**
- **Antimetabolites**
- **Antitumor antibiotics**

- **Hormones**
- **Radiation therapy**
- **Miscellaneous antineoplastic agents**

ALKYLATING AGENTS

Alkylating agents interfere with the function of cancer cells by attaching to the protein within them and altering their chemical composition. These agents are extremely toxic and cause very unpleasant and even dangerous side effects.

Conditions treated with alkylating agents include:

- Hodgkin's disease
- Lymphosarcomal leukemias

- Multiple myelomas

ANTIMETABOLITES

Antimetabolites adversely affect cancer cells by interfering in a particular phase of their metabolism. They can cause severe bone marrow depression, which may necessitate their withdrawal.

Conditions treated with antimetabolites include:

- Acute lymphocytic leukemia in children
- Uterine choriocarcinoma
- Lymphosarcoma
- Hodgkin's disease

- Carcinomas of the reproductive tract, pancreas, liver, and gastrointestinal tract
- Tumors of the head, neck, brain, and gallbladder

ANTITUMOR ANTIBIOTICS

Antitumor antibiotics interfere with the RNA synthesis of cancer cells or cause a split in the DNA chains of cancer cells. They should not be confused with anti-infective antibiotics as they do not have anti-infective properties.

Conditions treated by antitumor antibiotics include:

- Wilms' tumor
- Certain lymphomas
- Choriocarcinoma
- Hodgkin's disease
- Solid tumors of the breast, bone, bladder, lung, thyroid gland, and ovaries

- Ewing's sarcoma
- Adenocarcinoma of the stomach, pancreas, colon, and rectum
- Tumors of the head, neck, and cervix

HORMONES

Hormones have a number of uses in the treatment of cancer even though their action is not fully understood. Hormones have produced remissions of certain cancers. Sex hormones have provided palliative treatment for carcinomas of the reproductive tract.

Conditions treated with hormones include:

- Acute lymphocytic leukemia in children
- Carcinoma of the prostate
- Breast cancer in postmenopausal women
- Metastatic breast cancer

RADIATION THERAPY

Radiation is used to treat cancer; in fact, the majority of clients with cancer will receive some form of radiation therapy in addition to chemotherapy. Types of radiation therapy include external and internal therapy.

Conditions treated with external radiation therapy include:

- Salivary gland tumors
- Sarcomas
- Tumors of the lung and prostate

Conditions treated with internal radiation therapy include:

- Tumors of the prostate

MISCELLANEOUS ANTINEOPLASTIC AGENTS

Miscellaneous antineoplastic agents are a heterogeneous group of drugs having various active mechanisms. They include:

Vincristine sulfate (Oncovin)

Conditions treated with vincristine sulfate include:

- Acute leukemia

Vinblastine sulfate (Velban)

Conditions treated with vinblastine sulfate include:

- Choriocarcinoma
- Hodgkin's disease
- Lymphosarcoma

Procarbazine hydrochloride (Matulane)

Conditions treated with procarbazine hydrochloride include:

- Hodgkin's disease (orally)

Mechlorethamine hydrochloride (nitrogen mustard)

Conditions treated with mechlorethamine hydrochloride include:

- Chronic lymphocytic leukemia
- Polycythemia vera

Hydroxyurea (Hydrea)

Conditions treated with hydroxyurea include:

- Chronic granulocytic leukemia
- Malignant melanoma
- Ovarian carcinoma

Azathioprine (Imuran)

Conditions treated with azathioprine include:

- Rejection of kidney transplants

Mitotane (Lysodren)

Conditions treated with mitotane include:

- Adrenocortical carcinoma

Practice Test 2

Questions

2 - 1

Your client has cancer and is to receive a combination of fluorouracil (5-FU), levamisole, and leucovorin calcium. The client is also receiving allopurinol (Zyloprim). When teaching the client about 5-FU, you will include dermatological manifestations such as:

1. tearing, conjunctivitis, and blurred vision.
2. darkening of the skin along the veins and dark coloration of the nails.
3. rash, urticaria, and wheezing.
4. bone marrow suppression.

2 - 2

Your client has been diagnosed with leukemia. The client is to start vincristine (Oncovin) therapy. Your teaching plan will include which of the following information?

1. This drug is taken by mouth as home therapy.
2. This drug rarely affects coordination or mentation.
3. This drug may not be taken if the client is experiencing chickenpox or shingles.
4. This drug is not effective in the treatment of Hodgkin's disease.

2 - 3

A client's chemotherapy prescriptions include doxorubicin (Adriamycin) 20 mg per square meter (M_2) of body surface. The client's square meter area is 1.5. What is the correct dosage for this client?

1. 20 mg
2. 25 mg
3. 30 mg
4. 35 mg

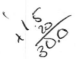

2 - 4

A client is to begin a regimen of fluorouracil (5-FU) following a mastectomy. You know the side effects of this medication may include:

1. constipation.
2. alopecia.
3. ventricular arrhythmias.
4. cystitis.

2 - 5

A 10-year-old client with acute lymphoblastic leukemia is to begin chemotherapy with methotrexate. You will teach the parents of the child that:

1. fluids are to be limited to 500 cc per day.
2. black, tarry stools are expected and of no concern.
3. blood work will be drawn periodically throughout the treatment course.
4. toothbrushing or rinsing should be limited to once daily.

2 - 6

During your clinical rotation in a cancer clinic, you will take special precautions when handling and mixing which of the following medications?

1. lorazepam (Ativan)
2. ranitidine (Zantac)
3. promethazine hydrochloride (Phenergan)
4. vinblastine sulfate

2 - 7

A client is receiving cyclophosphamide 600 mg, doxorubicin 50 mg, and vincristine sulfate 2 mg, intravenous chemotherapy protocol. Prior to administering chemotherapy, the nurse should first:

1. determine the presence of informed consent.
2. measure vital signs and determine height and weight.
3. ask the client what he knows about his condition.
4. inform the client of the side effects of the medications.

2 - 8

A client is receiving vincristine sulfate. When assessing the client, the nurse will know to:

1. note any changes in urinary patterns.
2. check skin surfaces for color changes.
3. ask the client for presence of metallic taste in mouth.
4. check hand grasps and deep tendon reflexes.

2 - 9

Your client has Stage III Hodgkin's disease. The client will receive intravenous chemotherapy with the medication mechlorethamine hydrochloride. To help control the side effects of this medication, you will:

✓ 1. administer an antiemetic before each treatment.
2. offer cool fluids daily.
3. make sure the room is cool and pleasant.
4. provide the client with small, frequent meals.

2 - 1 0

Your client is receiving cisplatin (Platinol AQ) following the removal of the right testis. You understand that the toxic effects of this drug include:

✓ 1. permanent hearing loss.
2. abdominal pain.
3. hyperpigmentation.
4. wheezing and crackles.

2 - 1 1

Your client is receiving nitrogen mustard, Oncovin, procarbazine, and prednisone (MOPP chemotherapy regimen) to treat Stage III Hodgkin's disease. You know the administration of this regimen is based on:

1. liver function.
2. respiratory status.
✓ 3. white blood cell values.
4. gastrointestinal status.

2 - 1 2

A client who is allergic to tartrazine is to begin treatment for lung cancer with the drug uracil mustard. You will:

1. chart the allergy and give the uracil mustard.
✓ 2. withhold the uracil mustard and notify the physician of the allergy.
3. administer a test dose of uracil mustard.
4. give the uracil mustard as prescribed.

2 - 1 3

Your client's daunorubicin (Cerubidine) infusion has infiltrated. You will discontinue the infusion and treat the extravasation site with:

1. warm compresses.
2. direct pressure.
3. the appropriate antidote.
4. ice packs.

2 - 1 4

You are giving ifosfamide (Ifex) to a client with testicular cancer. To prevent hemorrhagic cystitis, you will push fluids up to:

1. 1 liter daily.
2. 2 liters daily.
3. 3 liters daily.
4. 4 liters daily.

2 - 1 5

Your client is receiving high dosages of methotrexate to treat osteosarcoma. The drug leucovorin (folinic acid) has also been prescribed. You know the purpose of leucovorin in this situation is to:

1. facilitate the action of methotrexate.
2. destroy malignant cells.
3. serve as a palliative treatment.
4. minimize methotrexate toxicity.

2 - 1 6

A child with Wilms' tumor is receiving dactinomycin (Cosmegen). You learn that the child has contracted chickenpox. You will:

1. administer the medication as prescribed.
2. withhold the medication and notify the physician of the child's chickenpox.
3. document the client's chickenpox and give the varicella-zoster immunoglobulin (VZIG).
4. anticipate a prescription for an antiviral medication such as Famvir.

2 - 1 7

A client has stomatitis after a round of chemotherapy with cyclophosphamide (Cytoxan). To treat this condition, you teach the client to:

1. use a mouthwash containing alcohol after each meal.
2. limit smoking.
3. suck on ice chips periodically.
4. consume soft, bland foods.

2 - 1 8

A client is receiving docetaxel (Taxotere) to treat metastatic breast cancer. You will assess the client for evidence of myelosuppression such as:

1. asthenia.
2. anemia.
3. stomatitis.
4. alopecia.

2 - 1 9

Your client is receiving the myelosuppressive drug etoposide phosphate (Etopophos). You know that the client's greatest risk for infection occurs within:

1. the first week of administration.
2. 7 to 14 days following administration.
3. 14 to 28 days following administration.
4. 6 to 8 weeks following administration.

2 - 2 0

Clients receiving initial treatment with doxorubicin hydrochloride should be taught that:

1. urine may be dark green for 1 to 2 days.
2. hair growth will resume 1 to 2 months after the drug is stopped.
3. the drug may decrease urine concentration of uric acid.
4. immunizations should not be received during drug therapy.

2 - 2 1

You notice that crystals have formed in the intravenous infusion solution of fluorouracil (5-FU) you are preparing for your client. You will:

1. withhold the solution and notify the physician.
2. redissolve the crystals by warming.
3. recognize the crystals as normal and proceed with the infusion.
4. mix the solution with 0.9% NaCl to dissolve the crystals.

2 - 2 2

A client experiencing leukemia is receiving busulfan (Myleran) and has developed bone marrow suppression. Which nursing diagnosis has the highest priority?

1. activity intolerance
2. altered peripheral tissue perfusion
3. fluid volume deficit: Hemorrhage
4. infection

Practice Test 2

Answers, Rationales, and Explanations

2 - 1

② **Fluorouracil (5-FU) may cause darkening of the skin along the veins and dark coloration of the nails.**

1. Tearing, conjunctivitis, and blurred vision are side effects of the antineoplastic levamisole, not 5-FU. These side effects are not dermatological manifestations.

3. Rash and urticaria are side effects of leucovorin (antidote for methotrexate), not 5-FU.

4. Allopurinol (Zyloprim) may cause bone marrow suppression, which is not a dermatological manifestation.

Pregnancy Category: D
Client Need: Physiological Integrity

2 - 2

③ **Vincristine (Oncovin) should not be administered if the client has chickenpox or shingles because the immunosuppressant effect of this neoplastic medication may cause chickenpox or shingles to generalize and become more severe.**

1. Vincristine (Oncovin) is administered intravenously.

2. Vincristine (Oncovin) commonly causes peripheral neuropathy (pathology of the nerves).

4. The immunosuppressant effect of vincristine (Oncovin) has made it very useful in the treatment of Hodgkin's disease.

Pregnancy Category: D
Client Need: Health Promotion/Maintenance

2 - 3

③ **The correct dosage for this client is 30 mg.**
   Formula:
   Multiply 20 mg (dosage) by 1.5 square meters (M$_2$)
   20 mg $\times$ 1.5 M$_2$ = 30 mg

1 and 2. 20 mg and 25 mg are under dosages for this client's body surface.

4. 35 mg is an overdose for this client's body surface.

Pregnancy Category: D
Client Need: Safe, Effective Care Environment

2 - 4

② **Alopecia (hair loss) is a side effect of fluorouracil (5-FU) therapy. Fluorouracil is an antineoplastic agent whose impact on chromosomal structure contributes to numerous side effects, including: Nausea, vomiting, diarrhea, leukopenia (low white blood cell count), and alopecia.**

1. Fluorouracil (5-FU) may cause diarrhea, not constipation. Other gastrointestinal side effects include nausea, vomiting, and stomatitis.
3. Fluorouracil (5-FU) does not cause ventricular arrhythmias. It may cause hypotension and bradycardia.
4. Fluorouracil (5-FU) does not cause cystitis (inflammation of the urinary bladder), but it may cause urinary retention.

Pregnancy Category: D
Client Need: Physiological Integrity

2 - 5

③ **Blood work will be drawn periodically to assess the methotrexate's impact on blood counts and renal function. Methotrexate is an antimetabolite drug that has many potential side effects, including thrombocytopenia (decrease in platelets), renal impairment, anemia, and leukopenia (decrease in leukocytes).**

1. Fluids should be encouraged, not limited.
2. Black, tarry-looking stools are a reportable condition that could indicate gastrointestinal bleeding.
4. Oral care must be scrupulously maintained to help prevent stomatitis (inflammation of the mouth), which is a common side effect of antineoplastic agents.

Pregnancy Category: X
Client Need: Physiological Integrity

2 - 6

④ **Special precautions should be taken when handling vinblastine sulfate (Velban). Vinblastine sulfate (Velban) is an antineoplastic medication whose arrest of cell growth is dependent on blocking cell division. Because of its potent effect on mitosis, it has been associated with cancer risk for those exposed to the drug, including those who prepare the medication prior to its administration.**

1, 2, and 3. Lorazepam (Ativan), ranitidine (Zantac), and promethazine hydrochloride (Phenergan) have no documented risks for persons who handle them.

Pregnancy Category: C
Client Need: Safe, Effective Care Environment

2 - 7

① Before administering antineoplastic drugs, the nurse must know that the client has signed the Informed Consent form. Informed consent is an agreement by a client to accept a sequence of treatments/procedures following thorough explanation of the risks and other relevant facts.

2. Baseline data is essential before receiving any medication. However, clients do not need to sign an Informed Consent form before taking all medication. When receiving certain antineoplastic drugs, the client must sign the Informed Consent form.

3. Assessing a client's knowledge level about his condition is very helpful when caring for clients. However, it is not essential that the nurse determine the extent of the client's knowledge before administering antineoplastic drugs. It is essential to have the correct forms signed.

4. Informing clients of the side effects of drugs is part of the explanation that should be given in connection with the signing of the Informed Consent form.

Pregnancy Category: cyclophosphamide, C; doxorubicin, C; vincristine, D
Client Need: Safe, Effective Care Environment

2 - 8

④ The nurse will assess the client's hand grasps and deep tendon reflexes. Side effects of vincristine sulfate include peripheral neuropathies. Assessing hand grasps and deep tendon reflexes can help to determine if the client's sensorimotor functioning is intact.

1. Urinary pattern disturbances occur with Cytoxan and Adriamycin.

2. Fluorouracil (Efudex) may cause skin surface changes.

3. Metallic taste in mouth occurs with fluorouracil and cisplatin (Platinol AQ).

Pregnancy Category: D
Client Need: Physiological Integrity

2 - 9

① You will administer an antiemetic before each treatment. The side effects of mechlorethamine (Mustargen) include nausea and vomiting, which usually lasts from 12 to 24 hours.

2. Without antiemetics, the client may have difficulty keeping po fluids down.

3. Maintaining a cool environment is helpful when clients are subject to nausea and vomiting. However, antiemetics can help control nausea and vomiting.

4. It is advisable to serve small, frequent meals when clients are subject to nausea and vomiting. However, antiemetics can actually help control nausea and vomiting.

Pregnancy Category: D
Client Need: Physiological Integrity

2 - 1 0

(1) **Toxic effects of cisplatin include permanent hearing loss, tinnitus, and ototoxicity. Cisplatin is an alkylating agent that alters the chemical composition of protein.**

2, 3, and 4. Abdominal pain, hyperpigmentation, and crackles are not among the toxic effects of the drug cisplatin.

Pregnancy Category: D
Client Need: Health Promotion/ Maintenance

2 - 1 1

(3) **You know the administration of MOPP chemotherapy is based on white blood cell values. This combination of drugs can cause bone marrow suppression. Nitrogen mustard is an alkylating agent. Oncovin (vincristine sulfate) is a miscellaneous antineoplastic drug. Procarbazine hydrochloride is a miscellaneous antineoplastic drug. Prednisone is a corticosteroid hormonal drug. Prednisone is used more than any other hormone in treating malignancies.**

1. Liver function studies are not used to determine the administration of the MOPP regimen.

2 and 4. Side effects of the MOPP regimen do not include adverse respiratory or gastrointestinal findings.

Pregnancy Category: nitrogen mustard, Oncovin, and procarbazine, D; prednisone, C
Client Need: Physiological Integrity

2 - 1 2

(2) **The uracil mustard should be withheld and the physician notified if the client is allergic to tartrazine (a dye found in drug capsules). Uracil mustard is an alkylating agent, a derivative of nitrogen mustard used in treating certain types of tumors.**

1. The uracil mustard should not be given since the client is allergic to the tartrazine (dye found in the capsules).

3. A test dosage should not be given since you already know the client is allergic to the dye (tartrazine) found in the capsules.

4. The drug should not be given since the client is allergic to a dye (tartrazine) found in the capsules.

Pregnancy Category: D
Client Need: Health Promotion/Maintenance

2 - 1 3

④   Ice packs would be appropriate to treat extravasations associated with daunorubicin (Cerubidine). Cerubidine is an antibiotic antineoplastic drug used in the treatment of leukemias. You should observe for EKG changes, bone marrow suppression (low blood counts), hepatotoxicity, skin changes, and severe cellulitis (tissue sloughing).

1. Warm compresses would be appropriate to treat an extravasation of vinca alkaloid such as vincristine and vinblastine, not daunorubicin.

2. Direct pressure should not be applied. Direct pressure would further irritate the tissues that have been infiltrated.

3. There is no specific antidote for daunorubicin hydrochloride. Usually palliative treatments are given, such as ice packs.

Pregnancy Category: D

Client Need: Physiological Integrity

2 - 1 4

③   A minimum of 3 liters of fluid daily should be encouraged to prevent the potential for hemorrhagic cystitis.

1 and 2. One or two liters of fluid is not enough to prevent hemorrhagic cystitis when using the drug ifosfamide (Ifex).

4. Four liters is an unnecessarily high amount of fluid.

Pregnancy Category: D

Client Need: Health Promotion/Maintenance

2 - 1 5

④   The drug leucovorin is given to minimize methotrexate toxicity, such as bone marrow suppression and renal damage. When leucovorin is administered to minimize the toxic effects of methotrexate, the treatment is referred to as the leucovorin rescue. Methotrexate is an antimetabolite antineoplastic drug. It exerts its action by interfering with the formation of the reduced or active form of folic acid in the body.

1. Leucovorin (folinic acid) is not an antineoplastic drug and will not facilitate the action of methotrexate.

2. Leucovorin (folinic acid) is the calcium salt of folic acid that is used to antagonize the effects of methotrexate. It does not destroy cancer cells.

3. Leucovorin (folinic acid) is not used in the palliative treatment of osteosarcoma.

Pregnancy Category: methotrexate, X; leucovorin, C

Client Need: Physiological Integrity

2 - 1 6

② **Dactinomycin (Cosmegen) is contraindicated for clients who are infected with chicken-pox because of the risk of serious generalization of the chickenpox and possible death. Dactinomycin is an antibiotic antineoplastic drug. It exerts its effect by interfering with RNA synthesis.**

1. Continuing to give the dactinomycin (Cosmegen) could cause the chickenpox to generalize and lead to death.
3. Varicella-zoster immunoglobulin is given prophylactically to prevent chickenpox. This child already has chickenpox.
4. Famvir is an antiviral drug used to treat shingles.

Pregnancy Category: C

Client Need: Health Promotion/Maintenance

2 - 1 7

④ **Soft, bland foods that do not irritate the mucosa should be encouraged for people who have stomatitis.**

1. Mouthwashes containing alcohol should be avoided since they irritate the mucosa.
2. All smoking should be discouraged (not just limited) since it irritates the mucosa.
3. Extreme temperatures (cold/hot) should be avoided since they further traumatize the mucosa.

Pregnancy Category: D

Client Need: Physiological Integrity

2 - 1 8

② **You will assess for anemia. Myelosuppression inhibits bone marrow function (hematology).**

1. Asthenia (paresthesia) is an adverse reaction associated with the central nervous system, not the hematologic system.
3. Stomatitis (inflammation of the mouth) is associated with the gastrointestinal tract, not the hematologic system.
4. Alopecia (hair loss) is associated with the skin, not the hematologic system.

Pregnancy Category: D

Client Need: Physiological Integrity

2 - 1 9

② **You know the greatest risk of infection will occur within 7 to 14 days following the administration of the myelosuppressive drug etoposide phosphate (Etopophos). Myelosuppressants inhibit bone marrow function, which places clients receiving these agents in jeopardy of infection.**

1, 3, and 4. The greatest risk for infection occurs within 7 to 14 days following the administration of myelosuppressant drugs.

Pregnancy Category: D

Client Need: Health Promotion/Maintenance

2-20

④ **Clients receiving doxorubicin hydrochloride should not receive immunizations since their immune systems will be compromised.**

1. Urine may be red (not dark green) for 1 to 2 days during the initial therapy.
2. Hair growth will resume in 2 to 5 months (not 1 to 2 months) after the drug is stopped.
3. Doxorubicin may increase (not decrease) blood and urine concentrations of uric acid.

Pregnancy Category: D
Client Need: Health Promotion/Maintenance

2-21

② **Should crystals form in a solution of fluorouracil (5-FU), they should be redissolved by warming before administration.**

1. It is not necessary to withhold the solution. The crystals can be redissolved by warming.
3. Crystals are not normal and the solution should not be given until they have been redissolved by warming.
4. Fluorouracil (5-FU) can be given intravenously with 0.9% NaCl. However, this has nothing to do with redissolving crystals.

Pregnancy Category: Injection, D; topical form, X
Client Need: Safe, Effective Care Environment

2-22

④ **Infection, especially a viral infection, can be life threatening and therefore has the highest priority. Bone marrow is responsible for producing red and white blood cells. When bone marrow is suppressed, the client becomes open to infection and may experience anemia.**

1. Activity intolerance is not life threatening and can be treated with red blood cells. An increase in red blood cells will elevate energy levels.
2. Volume expanders can be administered when tissue perfusion is a problem.
3. In the event of fluid volume deficit, platelets can be administered.

Pregnancy Category: D
Client Need: Physiological Integrity

Practice Test 3

Cardiovascular Agents

OVERVIEW

Cardiovascular agents treat and/or prevent various conditions affecting the heart's ability to pump oxygenated blood to the tissues and provide the tissues with other nutrients. Cardiovascular agents also treat and/or prevent conditions affecting the removal of carbon dioxide and other waste products from the body.

Cardiovascular agents include:

- Antianginals
- Antiarrhythmics
- Antihypertensives
- Antilipemics
- Inotropics

ANTIANGINALS

Antianginals are vasodilating substances, such as nitrates and calcium channel blockers, that relax the smooth muscle layer of arterial blood vessels.

Conditions treated with antianginals include:

- Angina pectoris (acute)
- Angina pectoris (as a prophylaxis)

ANTIARRHYTHMICS

Antiarrhythmic substances are generally administered to treat clients with heart disease or a disease that affects cardiovascular function. Arrhythmias include any heart rate or rhythm other than the normal sinus rhythm.

Conditions treated with antiarrhythmics include:

- Atrial fibrillation
- Paroxysmal atrial tachycardia
- Premature ventricular contractions (PVC)
- Ventricular tachycardia

ANTIHYPERTENSIVES

Antihypertensives are administered to lower blood pressure. Many antihypertensives lower blood pressure by dilating arterial blood vessels. Dilating the arterial blood vessels will increase the amount of space available for the circulating blood. An increase in available space for circulating blood will lower blood pressure.

Conditions treated with antihypertensives include:

- Essential hypertension
- Hypertension (mild, moderate, severe)

ANTILIPEMICS

Antilipemics are used in conjunction with diet and exercise to reduce blood lipids (fats or fatlike substances in the blood).

Conditions treated with antilipemics include:

- Primary hypercholesterolemia
- Pruritus caused by partial bile obstruction

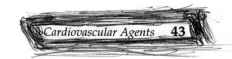

INOTROPICS (CARDIOTONIC SUBSTANCES)

Inotropics (cardiotonic substances) increase the force of contraction of the heart muscle (myocardium). As a result of the increased contractility of the myocardium, cardiac output is increased, blood flow to the kidneys and periphery is improved, venous pressure is improved, and excess fluid (edema) is excreted.

Conditions treated with inotropics (cardiotonic substances) include:

- Atrial fibrillation
- Atrial flutter
- Congestive heart failure
- Paroxysmal atrial tachycardia

Practice Test 3

Questions

3 - 1

A client arrives in the Emergency Department complaining of "crushing" chest pain. You anticipate a prescription for which of the following?

1. nifedipine (Procardia)
2. nizatidine (Axid)
3. nortriptyline hydrochloride
4. nystatin (Mycostatin)

3 - 2

A client's hypertension is to be treated with enalapril (Vasotec). The mechanism of action of this ACE inhibitor will:

1. increase renal excretion of sodium and water.
2. increase vasoconstriction.
3. inhibit the production of angiotensin II.
4. decrease heart rate and venous return.

3 - 3

Which of the following is a common early sign of digitalis toxicity?

1. tachycardia
2. constipation
3. dysrhythmia
4. anorexia

3 - 4

A client is taking the calcium channel blocker nifedipine (Procardia) for the control of moderate hypertension. The client is experiencing postural hypotension. Nursing interventions will include:

1. instructing your client not to lie on the left side.
2. increasing the calcium channel blocker dosage.
3. checking the blood pressure while the client is supine.
4. assisting the client in changing positions slowly.

3 - 5

A client is admitted to your unit in congestive heart failure. You are to administer digoxin 0.25 mg intravenously. The purpose of this medication is to:

1. decrease peripheral vascular resistance by vasodilation.
2. improve cardiac output and therefore renal perfusion.
3. increase heart rate and therefore cardiac output.
4. terminate paroxysmal atrial tachycardia.

3 - 6

Which of the following would be most important when teaching clients who are receiving a first prescription for prazosin (Minipress)?

1. Monitor their blood pressure.
2. Avoid sudden changes in position.
3. Take their medication at the same time each day whether it is morning or evening.
4. Consult a pharmacist before taking cold remedies.

3 - 7

A sympatholytic (beta-adrenergic blocking agent) atenolol (Tenormin) has been prescribed for a client with hypertension. Which question would be most appropriate for the nurse to ask the client before administering the first dosage?

1. "What kind of work do you do?"
2. "Are you allergic to fish or iodine?"
3. "Have you just eaten?"
4. "Do you have any respiratory problems?"

3 - 8

During admission assessment, your client tells you she takes quinidine 4 times a day. You know this medication:

1. is used in the treatment of malaria.
2. normally causes a widened QRS.
3. rarely causes toxic side effects.
4. is a Class I antiarrhythmic.

3 - 9

A client is on numerous medications following an acute myocardial infarction. The client is lethargic and has slurred speech. Which medication do you associate with these adverse reactions?

1. nitroglycerin infusion 5 mcg/min at increments q 3–5 min until response is noted
2. aspirin 325 mg by mouth, daily
3. lidocaine hydrochloride 4 mg/min continuous infusion
4. heparin sodium 800 units/h continuous infusion

3 - 1 0

A client is experiencing a hypertensive crisis. Blood pressure is 227/143 mmHg. Prescription reads: Diazoxide 100 mg intravenously. You know this medication will:

1. decrease the heart rate by vagal stimulation.
2. directly relax arteriolar smooth muscle.
3. promote diuresis.
4. block calcium channels.

3 - 1 1

Your client has elevated serum triglyceride levels and has started a regimen of clofibrate (Atromid-S) 500 mg by mouth every 4 hours. Regarding administration of this medication, you know that:

1. marked decreases in triglyceride levels are seen within 24 hours.
2. this medication is not indicated if triglyceride levels are > 500 mg/dl.
3. this medication has been used in the treatment of diabetes insipidus.
4. this medication may be used in hepatic failure.

3 - 1 2

Colestipol (Colestid), an antilipemic, acts by binding with bile acids. In addition to lowering cholesterol, there is a risk of decreasing the level of:

1. B complex vitamins.
2. fat-soluble vitamins.
3. serum potassium.
4. albumin.

3 - 1 3

A client is complaining of chest pain. An electrocardiogram (EKG) shows sinus bradycardia at 38 beats per minute with occasional premature ventricular contractions. The anticipated drugs of choice are:

1. oxygen and lidocaine.
2. oxygen and atropine.
3. lidocaine and morphine.
4. oxygen and verapamil.

3 - 1 4

A friend is hypertensive and has been on an angiotensin-converting enzyme (ACE) inhibitor for years. She calls to tell you she is pregnant. You encourage her to call her physician as soon as possible because she will soon need:

1. an increase in the angiotensin-converting enzyme.
2. a diuretic to work in combination with the angiotensin-converting enzyme inhibitor.
3. to discontinue the angiotensin-converting enzyme inhibitor.
4. to add a calcium channel blocker to the angiotensin-converting enzyme inhibitor.

3 - 1 5

The laboratory values for your client indicate a cholesterol level of 2246 mg/dl. You anticipate the administration of:

1. cholestyramine (Questran).
2. clofibrate (Atromid-S).
3. chloramphenicol (AK-Chlor).
4. chlortetracycline (Aureomycin).

3 - 1 6

Your client is to receive 0.125 mg digoxin by mouth daily. You would withhold the medication and notify the physician if the client had:

1. a headache and an apical pulse of 74 beats per minute.
2. an apical pulse of 92 beats per minute.
3. nausea and an apical pulse of 52 beats per minute.
4. leg cramps.

3 - 1 7

The physician has discontinued your client's nitroglycerin infusion and has placed the client on transdermal ointment 2%. Regarding the administration of this ointment, you know to:

1. cover the ointment with a transdermal nitroglycerin patch.
2. rub the ointment into the client's skin thoroughly.
3. apply the paste to the same area consistently.
4. check the client's blood pressure and pulse prior to application.

3 - 1 8

Your client has been discharged with a prescription for amlodipine besylate (Norvasc). You will include the following in your discharge instructions:

1. Medication may cause bradycardia.
2. Medication may cause a drop in blood pressure.
3. Medication cannot cause angina.
4. Medication is contraindicated while taking sublingual nitroglycerin.

3 - 1 9

Your client is admitted with the complaint of "fast, skipping heartbeats." The client is to receive disopyramide (Norpace) 200 mg every 6 hours by mouth. Because Norpace is available only in oral form, you know that:

1. it is not used in acute situations.
2. it must be taken with milk.
3. the onset of action is between 1 to 2 hours.
4. it must be given 30 minutes before or 1 hour after meals.

3 - 2 0

Your client has a 6 beat run of ventricular tachycardia. A lidocaine infusion was prescribed at 2 mg/min. The infusion is mixed with 2g/500 cc of lactated Ringer's solution. You will deliver:

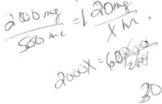

1. 3 cc per hour.
2. 6 cc per hour.
3. 30 cc per hour.
4. 60 cc per hour.

3 - 2 1

You observe an increase in your client's heart rate from 70 to 90 beats per minute to 120 beats per minute. The client is experiencing frequent multifocal premature ventricular contractions, many of which are paired. You are to give 50 mg of lidocaine (Zylocaine) intravenously, now. You know this medication was prescribed because it:

1. acts as a local anesthetic to the heart muscle.
2. is the treatment of choice for sinus tachycardia.
3. is a ventricular antiarrhythmic.
4. is an analgesic.

3 - 2 2

Your client was treated in the emergency department for intermittent atrial fibrillation and discharged with a prescription for digitoxin (Crystodigin). You will teach the client that:

1. digitoxin is interchangeable with digoxin.
2. digitoxin has a very short half-life and must be taken 4 times a day.
3. the average dosage of digitoxin is 3 to 5 mg daily.
4. digitoxin must be taken once daily.

3 - 2 3

Your client has edema secondary to congestive heart failure and has received furosemide (Lasix) 20 mg intravenously twice a day for the past 3 days. Appropriate nursing actions for this client would include:

1. Encourage intake of fluids by mouth.
2. Keep room dimly lit.
3. Monitor electrolytes.
4. Avoid/discourage high-potassium foods.

3 - 2 4

After you give your client a sublingual nitro-glycerin tablet, your client complains of a headache. You know this is:

1. considered an allergic reaction to nitro-glycerin.
2. unrelated to the nitroglycerin.
3. unlikely to get better even with smaller dosages of nitroglycerin.
4. a common side effect of nitroglycerin.

3 - 2 5

Your client is to be discharged from the Emergency Department after experiencing an anginal episode. When the client asks you what should be taken when chest pains are experienced at home, you tell the client to:

1. apply nitroglycerin ointment 1/2 inch.
2. apply a nitroglycerin transdermal patch 2.5 mg/24 hours.
3. take a nitroglycerin tablet 3 mg sublingually.
4. take a nitroglycerin tablet 0.3 mg sublingually.

3 - 2 6

A client with pheochromocytoma has a blood pressure of 268/180 mmHg. Which medication would be administered?

1. nitroprusside (Nitropress)
2. dopamine (Dopastat)
3. norepinephrine (Levophed)
4. ephedrine (Primatene)

3 - 2 7

A 5-year-old is hospitalized with congestive heart failure. Digoxin (Lanoxin) elixir is prescribed. The child weighs 44 pounds. The physician prescribes a maintenance dosage of 10 mcg/kg. Available is Lanoxin pediatric elixir 50 mcg/ml. The nurse will administer:

1. 2.6 ml.
2. 3.5 ml.
3. 4.2 ml.
4. 5.7 ml.

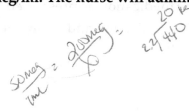

3-28

Your client had an acute myocardial infarction and is to be given atenolol (Tenormin) 5 mg intravenously stat. You know this medication will:

1. increase the heart rate.
2. reduce myocardial oxygen consumption.
3. increase the blood pressure.
4. lyse thrombus formation.

3-29

Your institution's premix of lidocaine infusion is 2 grams lidocaine per 500 cc of dextrose 5% in water. Your client is to have an infusion rate of 3 milligrams per minute. The infusion is running at 50 cc an hour. You will:

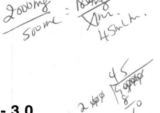

1. decrease the rate by 5 cc an hour.
2. increase the rate by 10 cc an hour.
3. leave the rate at 50 cc an hour.
4. withhold the infusion and consult with the physician.

3-30

A client with diabetes has developed hypertension and is receiving the angiotensin-converting enzyme (ACE) inhibitor enalapril (Vasotec). The client will need to be monitored for:

1. serum potassium depletion.
2. serum sodium depletion.
3. serum potassium elevation.
4. digoxin toxicity.

3-31

A client on telemetry is receiving several medications, including a prescription for the calcium channel blocker diltiazem (Cardizem CD) 30 mg by mouth, 3 times a day. The electrocardiogram on telemetry shows a second-degree AV block, Type II, with a rate of 48. You will:

1. assess blood pressure.
2. monitor apical pulse rate.
3. give the medication as prescribed.
4. hold the medication and notify the physician.

3 - 3 2

Phentolamine mesylate (Regitine) is administered for the treatment of hypertension
associated with pheochromocytoma. Because
of its vasodilatory effect, it is also administered via the subcutaneous route to treat:

1. second-degree burns.
2. norepinephrine extravasations.
3. fungal infections of the oral mucosa.
4. subcutaneous emphysema.

3 - 3 3

You are to administer procainamide
(Pronestyl-SR) 500 mg by mouth. For which
of the following conditions will you withhold the dosage and notify the physician?

1. serum glucose of 115 mg/dl
2. blood pressure (systolic) of 138 mmHg
3. apical pulse of 42 beats per minute
4. blood pressure (diastolic) of 72 mmHg

3 - 3 4

During the cardiopulmonary resuscitation of
your client, the code team requests an
epinephrine infusion 2 mcg/min. In the
crash cart you find a 1-ml vial of a 1:1000
epinephrine solution and a 500-ml bag of
normal saline. You will:

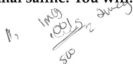

1. mix 1 vial in the 500-ml bag and infuse at 6 cc an hour.
2. mix 0.5 ml of the epinephrine in the bag and infuse at 6 cc an hour.
3. mix the 1-ml vial in the 500-ml normal saline and infuse at 60 cc an hour.
4. question the request because this is an excessive amount of medication.

3 - 3 5

Your client is anxious and tells you, "My
heart is racing." An electrocardiogram shows
a supraventricular tachycardia at 198 beats
per minute. Which medication do you
anticipate administering?

1. adenosine 6 mg by mouth
2. adenosine 6 mg intravenously
3. atropine 1 mg by mouth
4. atropine 1 mg intravenously

3 - 3 6

Your client is to be discharged today and has a prescription for nitroglycerin 0.4-mg tablets, sublingual, as needed. You will instruct your client to:

1. swallow the tablets whole if chest pain occurs.
2. take at least 4 tablets before seeking medical help for chest pain.
3. refill the prescription annually to ensure freshness.
4. discard the cotton inside the medication bottle.

3 - 3 7

Your client is receiving a loading dose of digoxin 0.5 mg po in divided dosages over a 24-hour period. You will recognize the most common and earliest adverse reaction to digoxin as:

1. paresthesia.
2. nausea and anorexia.
3. dry eyes.
4. dizziness and vertigo.

3 - 3 8

Your client is receiving warfarin (Coumadin) following an episode of thrombophlebitis and is to be discharged on this medication. You will instruct your client to:

1. wear pants with an elastic waistband.
2. avoid crossing the legs.
3. consume foods high in vitamin K.
4. use birth control pills to prevent pregnancy.

3 - 3 9

A client has ingested too many "diet pills" containing amphetamines. You will monitor the client for which common side effect?

1. hypotension
2. sedation
3. tachyarrhythmias
4. euphoria

3-40

A client experiencing chest pains and anterior myocardial infarction begins to show frequent multifocal premature ventricular contractions (PVCs) on his EKG. Which medication do you anticipate delivering?

1. atropine sulfate
2. adenosine
3. lidocaine 2 mg po
4. lidocaine 2 mg/min by continuous infusion

3-41

You administer a propranolol hydrochloride (Inderal) 80-mg extended-release capsule daily to treat a client experiencing angina pectoris. Upon discharge, you will teach the client to:

1. take the drug on an empty stomach.
2. discontinue taking the drug and notify the physician should constipation occur.
3. take the drug even when feeling well.
4. avoid prolonged exposure to the sun and wear protective clothing.

Practice Test 3

Answers, Rationales, and Explanations

3 - 1

① **You will anticipate a prescription for nifedipine (Procardia). Procardia is a calcium channel blocker that has coronary vasodilatory action. Vasodilation allows more oxygen to travel to the myocardial cells, thus relieving pain associated with ischemia (lack of oxygen). Procardia is administered for the treatment of angina pectoris (chest pain) caused by coronary insufficieny or vasospasm.**

2. Nizatidine (Axid) is an antiulcer agent and has no impact on chest pain.

3. Nortriptyline hydrochloride is a tricyclic antidepressant and has no impact on chest pain.

4. Nystatin (Mycostatin) is an antifungal agent and has no impact on chest pain.

Pregnancy Category: C

Client Need: Physiological Integrity

3 - 2

③ **Enalapril (Vasotec) inhibits production of angiotensin II, a potent vasoconstrictor. Enalapril (Vasotec) is an angiotensin-converting enzyme (ACE) inhibitor that inhibits conversion of angiotensin I to angiotensin II and lowers blood pressure by vasodilation.**

1. Angiotensin-converting enzyme (ACE) inhibitors are not diuretics; however, they indirectly increase fluid and sodium excretion by lowering the blood pressure.

2. Angiotensin-converting enzyme (ACE) inhibitors are vasodilators, not vasoconstrictors.

4. Angiotensin-converting enzymes (ACE) inhibitors have no direct cardiac effect.

Pregnancy Category: First trimester, C; Second trimester, D

Client Need: Physiological Integrity

3 - 3

④ **Anorexia is a common early sign of digitalis toxicity. Visual symptoms are also common early signs of toxicity and include colored halos around bright or green lights and a green or yellow tint to white objects.**

1. Tachycardia is usually a later sign of digitalis toxicity.

2. Constipation is not usually a sign of digitalis toxicity.

3. Dysrhythmia is usually a later sign of digitalis toxicity.

Pregnancy Category: C

Client Need: Physiological Integrity

3 - 4

④ **Clients experiencing postural hypotension should be assisted in changing positions slowly. Postural hypotension is a drop in blood pressure when a client's position is changed quickly from supine (lying on the back) to standing. Postural hypotension may cause syncope ("passing out"). Changing positions gradually helps avoid this and will prevent injury from a fall.**

1.   There is no reason why clients taking antihypertensives cannot lie on their left sides.

2.   Since hypotension has occurred, the dosage of Procardia may need to be decreased, not increased.

3.   Blood pressure should be checked while the client is lying, sitting, and standing to identify any drop in blood pressure (postural hypotension), not just when the client is supine.

Pregnancy Category: C

Client Need: Safe, Effective Care Environment

3 - 5

② **Digoxin improves cardiac output and therefore renal perfusion. Digoxin is a cardiac glycoside that has positive inotropic action (increases the force of the heart's contraction). This increased force of contraction improves tissue perfusion, improves cardiac filling time, and thus relieves congestive heart failure. Digoxin also lowers the heart rate, which increases the heart's resting time.**

1.   Digoxin is not a peripheral vasodilatory drug.

3.   Digoxin lowers the heart rate. It does not increase the heart rate.

4.   There is no indication that this client is experiencing atrial tachycardia.

Pregnancy Category: C

Client Need: Health Promotion/Maintenance

3 - 6

② **Clients receiving a first prescription for prazosin (Minipress) should avoid sudden changes in position. Prazosin (Minipress) is an antihypertensive. Orthostatic hypotension is a key side effect that should be monitored (especially early in treatment) since prazosin (Minipress) is an alpha-adrenergic blocker and has vasodilatory effects.**

1.   Monitoring the blood pressure is important but not the priority during the initial administration of this medication.

3.   Prazosin (Minipress) may cause drowsiness and should be administered in the evening.

4.   Consulting a pharmacist before taking cold remedies is important since many cold remedies cause sedation. However, changing positions slowly is the priority during the initial administration of this medication.

Pregnancy Category: C

Client Need: Safe, Effective Care Environment

3 - 7

④ **Clients receiving their first dosage of atenolol (Tenormin) should be asked if they have any respiratory problems. Atenolol (Tenormin) may cause bronchospasm and bronchoconstriction. A history of asthma, obstructive lung disease, or reactive airway disease could indicate a need to reexamine the appropriateness of administering beta-adrenergic blocking agents such as Tenormin.**

1. There are very few side effects of atenolol (Tenormin) that would interfere with work. Therefore, asking what kind of work the client does is not relevant.

2. Allergies to fish or iodine will not prohibit the taking of beta-blockers.

3. Beta-adrenergic blocking agents are usually not given specifically in reference to meals or the fullness or emptiness of the stomach.

Pregnancy Category: C

Client Need: Physiological Integrity

3 - 8

④ **Quinidine is a Class I antiarrhythmic. It is indicated for atrial, interatrial, and ventricular arrhythmias.**

1. Quinine is used in the treatment of malaria, not quinidine.

2. A wide QRS is not normal and might indicate quinidine toxicity.

3. Quinidine has numerous side effects and serum levels should be monitored.

Pregnancy Category: C

Client Need: Physiological Integrity

3 - 9

③ **Lidocaine hydrochloride is an antiarrhythmic drug whose toxic or adverse reactions include central nervous system symptoms such as lethargy, confusion, drowsiness, and slurred speech.**

1. Nitroglycerin may cause hypotension and headache, not lethargy and slurred speech.

2. Aspirin may cause gastrointestinal distress or bleeding, not lethargy and slurred speech.

4. Heparin sodium is an anticoagulant and may cause bleeding, not lethargy and slurred speech.

Pregnancy Category: B

Client Need: Physiological Integrity

3 - 1 0

② **Diazoxide (Hyperstat) is an antihypertensive (vasodilator) whose action directly relaxes arteriolar smooth muscles to lower blood pressure.**

1. Diazoxide does not affect the vagus nerve.
3. Diazoxide is not a diuretic.
4. Diazoxide is not a calcium channel blocker.

Pregnancy Category: C
Client Need: Physiological Integrity

3 - 1 1

③ **Clofibrate (Atromid-S) is an antilipemic and has been used investigationally to treat diabetes insipidus.**

1. It usually takes several days to see any changes in triglyceride levels once antilipemic therapy is begun and 3 weeks for peak effects.
2. Clofibrate (Atromid-S) is indicated for extreme elevations of triglycerides such as levels > 500 mg/dl. The normal triglyceride level for men is 40 to 160 mg/dl. The normal triglyceride level for women is 35 to 135 mg/dl.
4. Clofibrate (Atromid-S) should not be used during hepatic failure.

Pregnancy Category: C
Client Need: Physiological Integrity

3 - 1 2

② **The fat-soluble vitamins A, D, E, and K may also be excreted along with bile acids during antilipemic therapy.**

1. B complex vitamins and the other water-soluble vitamins are affected very little by colestipol (Colestid).
3. Serum potassium is affected little by colestipol (Colestid).
4. Albumin levels are affected very little by colestipol (Colestid).

Pregnancy Category: NR
Client Need: Physiological Integrity

3 - 1 3

② **The drugs of choice are oxygen and atropine. Atropine is the drug of choice for symptomatic bradycardia. It increases the conduction rate of the heart through the atrioventricular node (AV). Supplemental oxygen is also indicated to avoid myocardial ischemia.**

1. Lidocaine is not recommended to treat escape premature ventricular contractions (PVCs) associated with bradycardia. Premature ventricular contractions during bradycardia many times contribute to cardiac output.

3. The administration of morphine could potentiate bradycardia and would be contraindicated.

4. Verapamil would decrease the heart rate even more because it is a calcium channel blocker, which decreases cardiac contractibility.

Pregnancy Category: C
Client Need: Physiological Integrity

3 - 1 4

③ **She will need to discontinue the angiotensin-converting enzyme inhibitors. Angiotensin-converting enzyme inhibitors prevent the conversion of angiotensin I to angiotensin II (an endogenous vasoconstrictor). Because of their potentially adverse effects on the fetus, angiotensin-converting enzyme inhibitors are usually not given during pregnancy.**

1, 2, and 4. Angiotensin-converting enzyme inhibitors are usually contraindicated during pregnancy due to the medication's impact on circulation and enzyme conversion.

Pregnancy Category: First trimester, C; Second and third trimesters, D
Client Need: Safe, Effective Care Environment

3 - 1 5

② **When a client's cholesterol level is extremely high, a prescription for clofibrate (Atromid-S) is anticipated. The normal serum cholesterol level is 120 to 200 mg/dl depending on age and sex. Two grams of Atromid-S by mouth in divided dosages are usually prescribed to manage this condition. Although the mechanism is not clearly understood, this medication directly depresses the synthesis of cholesterol.**

1. Cholestyramine (Questran) is prescribed to treat moderate cholesterol levels.

3. Chloramphenicol (AK-Chlor) is an anti-infective and does not affect cholesterol levels.

4. Chlortetracycline (Aureomycin) is a bacteriostatic agent and does not affect cholesterol levels.

Pregnancy Category: C
Client Need: Physiological Integrity

3 - 1 6

③ **Digoxin should be withheld when a client experiences nausea and has a pulse rate below 60 beats per minute. Digoxin is a cardiotonic that strengthens the force of the myocardial contraction and slows the heart's rate. Toxic serum levels of this medication produce signs and symptoms including nausea, vomiting, bradyarrhythmia (heart rate less than 60 beats per minute), and visual disturbances.**

1. Headaches are not typically associated with elevated serum digoxin levels.
2. The dosage is usually withheld for heart rates < 60 or > 100 beats per minute.
4. Leg cramps are not associated with elevated serum digoxin levels.

Pregnancy Category: C

Client Need: Physiological Integrity

3 - 1 7

④ **Clients receiving nitroglycerin should have their blood pressure and pulse assessed prior to administration. Nitroglycerin is a vasodilatory drug available in tablet, capsule, spray, patch, ointment, or intravenous infusion form. Because of its vasodilatory action, hypotension may occur.**

1. Covering the nitroglycerin ointment with a nitroglycerin transdermal patch would be double dosing. The ointment could be covered with an occlusive dressing if prescribed.
2. Nitroglycerin ointment should not be rubbed or massaged into the client's skin; doing so will increase absorption and interfere with the sustained action of the medication.
3. To prevent skin irritation, topical sites should be rotated.

Pregnancy Category: C

Client Need: Health Promotion/Maintenance

3 - 1 8

② **Amlodipine besylate (Norvasc) may cause a drop in blood pressure. Amlodipine besylate is an antihypertensive and antianginal medication. It decreases myocardial contractibility and oxygen demand by inhibiting the transport of calcium ions into myocardial and smooth muscle cells. It is important to teach clients about potential postural hypotension and measures that avoid syncope or faintness that may occur with sudden position changes.**

1. Amlodipine besylate (Norvasc) may cause palpitations that are perceptible to the client, not bradycardia.
3. Amlodipine besylate (Norvasc) can cause angina.
4. Amlodipine besylate (Norvasc) causes a decrease in frequency and severity of angina attacks because of its coronary vasodilatory effects.

Pregnancy Category: C

Client Need: Health Promotion/Maintenance

3 - 1 9

① Disopyramide (Norpace) is available only in oral form and is therefore not used in acute situations. Disopyramide (Norpace) blocks sodium channels (local anesthetic effect) and slows conduction of electrical impulses in the heart. It is used to treat ectopic ventricular beats. Side effects include hypotension, congestive heart failure, worsened or new arrhythmias, nausea, and vomiting.

2. Disopyramide (Norpace) should not be taken with food because food may affect absorption.

3. The onset of action of disopyramide (Norpace) is 0.5 to 3.5 hours. Plasma levels peak within 2 to 2.5 hours and the effects persist for 1.5 to 8.5 hours after the last dose.

4. Disopyramide (Norpace) should be given on an empty stomach 1 hour before meals or 2 hours after meals.

Pregnancy Category: C
Client Need: Physiological Integrity

3 - 2 0

③ **30 cc per hour will be delivered.**

$$\frac{60 \text{ min}}{1 \text{ h}} \times \frac{2 \text{ mg}}{1 \text{ min}} \times \frac{1 \text{ q}}{1000 \text{ mg}} \times \frac{500 \text{ cc}}{2 \text{ gm}} = \textbf{30 cc per hour}$$

1, 2, and 4 are incorrect amounts.

Pregnancy Category: B
Client Need: Physiological Integrity

3 - 2 1

③ **Lidocaine (Zylocaine) is an antiarrhythmic when administered intravenously. When administered locally, it is an anesthetic. Because of lidocaine's impact on ventricular irritability, it is one of the drugs of choice for the treatment of premature ventricular contractions.**

1. The prescribed dosage and route of lidocaine (Zylocaine) indicates it is being given to treat ventricular antiarrhythmias, not for its anesthetic effects. Given locally, lidocaine acts as an anesthetic.

2. Lidocaine (Zylocaine) does not have an impact on sinus tachycardia.

4. Lidocaine (Zylocaine) is an analgesic only when administered locally.

Pregnancy Category: B
Client Need: Physiological Integrity

3 - 2 2

④ **Digitoxin must be taken on a once-daily schedule. The serum level of digitoxin should not fluctuate too widely. Digitoxin, like digoxin, has a relatively narrow therapeutic range, making it very important to take prescribed dosages on schedule. Erratic administration can quickly lead to serum levels outside the therapeutic range, which could cause arrhythmias. The normal serum digitoxin level is 20 to 30 mg/ml.**

1. Digitoxin and digoxin are not interchangeable.
2. Digitoxin has a longer half-life than digoxin.
3. The average adult dosage of digitoxin is 0.05 to 0.3 mg daily.

Pregnancy Category: C
Client Need: Health Promotion/Maintenance

3 - 2 3

③ **You will monitor electrolytes because potassium and sodium will be excreted in the urine. Furosemide (Lasix) is a loop diuretic (increases the secretion of urine) prescribed to manage edema associated with congestive heart failure.**

1. This client is receiving a diuretic. Encouraging fluid intake would be contraindicated.
2. Photosensitivity is a side effect of furosemide (Lasix), but it is not necessary to keep the client's room dimly lit.
4. Persons on loop diuretics are at risk for hypokalemia (potassium depletion in the circulating blood) and should consume foods high in potassium, such as bananas, broccoli, spinach, and navy beans.

Pregnancy Category: C
Client Need: Health Promotion/Maintenance

3 - 2 4

④ **Headache, dizziness, hypotension, and flushing are all common side effects of nitroglycerin and are due to the vasodilatory action of the drug.**

1. A headache is considered a side effect, not an allergic reaction to nitroglycerin.
2. Headache is directly related to the nitroglycerin's vasodilatory action.
3. Headache may be managed with smaller dosages of nitroglycerin.

Pregnancy Category: C
Client Need: Physiological Integrity

3 - 2 5

④ **Sublingual nitroglycerin is effective in relieving acute chest pain. Nitroglycerin (an antianginal agent) dilates coronary vessels and reduces oxygen demand on the myocardium. During acute angina, the sublingual route is quick and effective. Dosages of sublingual tablets are generally 0.3 mg, 0.4 mg, or 0.6 mg.**

1 and 2. Nitroglycerin ointment and nitroglycerin transdermal patches are usually prescribed for maintenance or prophylaxis of angina.

3.   Three mg is an excessive sublingual dosage and should not be taken.

Pregnancy Category: C

Client Need: Health Promotion/Maintenance

3 - 2 6

① **Nitroprusside (Nitropress) should be administered. Pheochromocytoma is a tumor that produces catecholamines and causes paroxysmal (sudden attacks of) hypertension in approximately 50% of clients. Nitroprusside (Nitropress) is an antihypertensive medication that has a vasodilatory effect. Because the client's blood pressure is extremely elevated, treatment of hypertension is imperative. Prolonged hypertension could result in a cerebrovascular accident (stroke).**

2, 3, and 4. Dopamine (Dopastat), norepinephrine (Levophed), and ephedrine (Primatene) would be contraindicated. They are all vasopressors (cause contraction of the muscles of capillaries and arteries) and would increase blood pressure further by stimulating adrenergic receptors.

Pregnancy Category: C

Client Need: Physiological Integrity

3 - 2 7

③ **The nurse will administer 4.2 ml of digoxin (Lanoxin) elixir. Converting the child's weight to kilograms: Approximately 21 kg (weight conversion: 2.2 pounds = 1 kg, 44/2.2 = approximately 21 kg). The child's digoxin dosage, based upon the child's weight, is 210 micrograms (21 kg x mcg/kg.)**

Calculation: 50 mcg/ml = 210 mcg/X ml

50X = 210

X = 4.2 ml

1, 2, and 4 are incorrect calculations.

Pregnancy Category: C

Client Need: Physiological Integrity

3 - 2 8

② **Atenolol (Tenormin) reduces myocardial oxygen demand. It is a beta-adrenergic blocker and affects the sympathetic nervous system by decreasing heart rate, blood pressure, and myocardial oxygen demand.**

1. Atenolol will decrease heart rate, not increase it.
3. Atenolol will decrease blood pressure, not increase it.
4. Atenolol is a beta-adrenergic blocker, not a thrombolytic.

Pregnancy Category: C
Client Need: Physiological Integrity

3 - 2 9

① **You will decrease the rate by 5 cc an hour.**

$$\frac{60 \text{ min}}{1 \text{ h}} \times \frac{3 \text{ mg}}{1 \text{ min}} \times \frac{1 \text{ gm}}{1000 \text{ mg}} \times \frac{500 \text{ cc}}{2 \text{ gm}} = \frac{45 \text{ cc}}{1 \text{ h}}$$

Formula:
2. To increase the rate by 10 cc an hour would infuse 60 cc an hour.
3. To leave the rate at 50 cc an hour would infuse 5 cc more an hour than prescribed.
4. The infusion is needed. It is the dosage that requires adjustment. There is no need to consult with the physician.

Pregnancy Category: B
Client Need: Safe, Effective Care Environment

3 - 3 0

③ **Serum potassium levels should be monitored when clients are receiving ACE inhibitors. Enalapril (Vasotec) is an angiotensin-converting enzyme (ACE) inhibitor. Its actions cause vasodilation in the treatment of hypertension. Potassium elevation (hyper-kalemia) is always a risk for clients who may have renal function deficits because the excretion of potassium is limited. Angiotensin-converting enzyme (ACE) inhibitors tend to augment this tendency.**

1. The angiotensin-converting enzyme (ACE) inhibitor enalapril (Vasotec) is not a diuretic and therefore does not deplete potassium.
2. Angiotensin-converting enzyme (ACE) inhibitors increase sodium and fluid excretion.
4. There is no indication that this client is receiving digoxin.

Pregnancy Category: First trimester, C; Second trimester, D
Client Need: Health Promotion/Maintenance

3 - 3 1

④ **The diltiazem (Cardizem CD) should be held and the physician notified. Diltiazem is a calcium channel blocker, antianginal, and coronary vasodilator. Diltiazem is contraindicated for marked bradyarrhythmias because the blocking of calcium channels decreases myocardial contractibility and will therefore worsen the bradyarrhythmia.**

1. More needs to be done than just assessing the client's blood pressure. The medication should be held.

2. The medication should be held and the physician notified, since giving the drug would worsen the bradyarrhythmia. Simply monitoring the apical pulse rate would not do anything to reverse the bradycardia.

3. The medication should be held and the physician notified. If the medication is administered, it will cause the client's heart rate to drop further.

Pregnancy Category: C

Client Need: Health Promotion/Maintenance

3 - 3 2

② **Phentolamine mesylate (Regitine) may be prescribed to treat norepinephrine extravasations (escape of norepinephrine into the tissues). Administration of phentolamine is the recommended treatment for damage of surrounding tissue associated with norepinephrine extravasation. Because norepinephrine (Levophed) has potent vasoconstrictive effects, tissue ischemia and necrosis may occur if infiltration occurs. The vasodilatory effect of phentolamine helps prevent such tissue damage.**

1. Second-degree burns are usually treated with anti-infectives.

3. Fungal infections of the oral mucosa are treated with antifungals.

4. Subcutaneous emphysema is often treated without pharmaceuticals.

Pregnancy Category: C

Client Need: Physiological Integrity

3 - 3 3

③ **Pronestyl-SR should be withheld and the physician notified if the client's apical pulse is 60 bpm or less. Procainamide (Pronestyl-SR) is an antiarrhythmic drug used to treat both atrial and ventricular arrhythmias. Signs of toxicity include electrocardiogram (ECG) changes, hypotension, and bradyarrhythmias (heart rate 60 bpm or less).**

1. The normal blood glucose level is 60 to 115 mg/dl. Since the client's serum glucose is 115 mg/dl, there is no reason to take any action.

2. A systolic blood pressure of 138 mmHg is expected in this situation.

4. A diastolic blood pressure of 72 mmHg is expected in this situation.

Pregnancy Category: C

Client Need: Physiological Integrity

3 - 3 4

③   Mix the 1-ml vial in the 500-ml normal saline and run at 60 cc an hour. Formula:

$$\frac{60 \text{ min}}{1 \text{ h}} \times \frac{2 \text{ mcg}}{1 \text{ min}} \times \frac{1 \text{ mg}}{1000 \text{ mcg}} \times \frac{500 \text{ cc}}{1 \text{ mg}} = 60 \text{ cc an hour}$$

Epinephrine (a sympathomimetic) may be used to restore cardiac rhythm in cardiac arrest.

1 and 2 are incorrect calculations.

4.   The request is appropriate and should not be questioned.

Pregnancy Category: C

Client Need: Physiological Integrity

3 - 3 5

②   You will anticipate giving adenosine (Adenocard) 6 mg intravenously. Because of its extremely short half-life, adenosine must be given in rapid intravenous boluses in dosages of 6 mg or 12 mg per bolus. Adenosine (Adenocard) is an antiarrhythmic medication whose tendency to slow conduction makes it a treatment of choice in supraventricular tachyarrhythmias.

1.   Adenosine is not given orally.

3 and 4. Atropine is used to treat bradyarrhythmias, not tachycardia.

Pregnancy Category: C

Client Need: Physiological Integrity

3 - 3 6

④   The cotton inside the medication bottle absorbs the drug and should be removed. Also, the medication should be kept in a dark-colored glass container because plastic absorbs it and light compromises the potency of the drug.

1.   Sublingual nitroglycerin tablets are to be held under the tongue or in the buccal pouch.

2.   It is usually recommended that clients seek medical help when 3 tablets taken at 5-minute intervals have not alleviated the chest pain.

3.   The prescription should be refilled every 3 to 6 months to maintain potency.

Pregnancy Category: C

Client Need: Health Promotion/Maintenance

3 - 3 7

② **Nausea, vomiting, and anorexia are common early adverse reactions to digoxin (Lanoxin) administration.**

1. Paresthesia (a sensation of numbness or tingling) is an uncommon adverse reaction to digoxin (Lanoxin) administration.

3. Dry eyes is an uncommon adverse reaction to digoxin (Lanoxin) administration. However, yellow-green halos around images, flashes of light, diplopia (double vision), and photophobia (unusual intolerance of light) are common adverse reactions.

4. Dizziness and vertigo are adverse reactions; however, they are not early reactions.

Pregnancy Category: C
Client Need: Physiological Integrity

3 - 3 8

② **Clients with thrombophlebitis should avoid crossing their legs because this places weight on the popliteal space and decreases venous return to the heart.**

1. Clients with thrombophlebitis should be instructed that constrictive garments like pants with elastic waistbands and girdles are contraindicated.

3. Warfarin (Coumadin) is an anticoagulant. Clients should be taught to avoid foods high in vitamin K because vitamin K impairs anticoagulation. Also, because warfarin (Coumadin) is an anticoagulant, clients should be assessed for hematuria.

4. Birth control pills are contraindicated for clients with a history of thrombophlebitis since they increase the risk of clot formation.

Pregnancy Category: X
Client Need: Physiological Integrity

3 - 3 9

③ **Clients taking amphetamines should be monitored carefully for tachyarrhythmias. Amphetamines are central nervous system (CNS) stimulants whose side effects include tachyarrhythmias, nervousness, sleeplessness, and loss of appetite.**

1 and 2. Hypotension and sedation are associated with the effects of sedatives and hypnotics, not stimulants like amphetamines.

4. Euphoria may occur; however, it is not a common side effect of amphetamines.

Pregnancy Category: C
Client Need: Health Promotion/Maintenance

3 - 4 0

④ **You will anticipate giving lidocaine 2 mg/min by continuous infusion. Lidocaine hydrochloride is an antiarrhythmic medication whose impact on ventricular arrhythmias is due to its suppression of automaticity (automatic action) and excitability of the myocardium. It may be given as a loading dose bolus, then by continuous infusion. It is not given orally.**

1. Atropine sulfate is used to treat bradyarrhythmias.
2. Adenosine is used to treat supraventricular tachyarrhythmias.
3. Lidocaine is not given in pill form.

Pregnancy Category: B
Client Need: Physiological Integrity

3 - 4 1

③ **You will teach the client to continue taking the drug even when feeling well. Propranolol hydrochloride (Inderal) should not be discontinued suddenly because doing so can exacerbate an angina attack and precipitate a myocardial infarction.**

1. Propranolol hydrochloride should be taken with food because it increases absorption of the drug.
2. Propranolol hydrochloride can cause constipation. However, the constipation can be treated with laxatives. Suddenly discontinuing the drug can cause attacks of angina and even precipitate a myocardial infarction.
3. Propranolol hydrochloride does not cause photosensitivity. There is no need to avoid sunlight or wear protective clothing.

Pregnancy Category: C
Client Need: Health Promotion/Maintenance

Practice Test 4

Fluid and Electrolytic Agents

OVERVIEW

Fluid and electrolytic agents magnify the ability of the renal system to selectively excrete electrolytes and water. They replace lost electrolytes and maintain the body's acid/base balance.

Fluid and electrolytic agents include:

- Acidifiers and alkalinizers
- Antidiuretics
- Diuretics
- Electrolytes and electrolyte modifiers

ACIDIFIERS AND ALKALINIZERS

ACIDIFIERS increase the acidity of substances to which they are added or exposed.

Acidifiers include:

- Ammonium chloride

Conditions treated with acidifiers include:

- Metabolic alkalosis

ALKALINIZERS increase the alkalinity of substances to which they are either added or exposed.

Alkalinizers include:

- Sodium bicarbonate
- Sodium lactate
- Tromethamine

Conditions treated with alkalinizers include:

- Metabolic acidosis
- Metabolic acidosis associated with cardiac bypass surgery

ANTIDIURETICS

Antidiuretics decrease urinary output by suppressing the rate of urine formation or by promoting the reabsorption of water. Hormones such as vasopressin regulate the reabsorption of water by the kidneys. Vasopressin is secreted by the posterior pituitary gland when body fluids must be conserved.

Conditions treated with vasopressin and its derivatives include:

- Diabetes insipidus
- Postoperative distention

DIURETICS

Diuretics facilitate the excretion of water and electrolytes from the body and thereby reduce the amount of excess fluid in the tissues. Diuretics include thiazides, loop diuretics, osmotic diuretics, and potassium-sparing diuretics.

Conditions treated with diuretics include:

- Endocrine disorders
- Heart failure
- Kidney and liver disease

ELECTROLYTES AND ELECTROLYTE MODIFIERS

Electrolytes disunite, or separate, into ions (particles carrying an electric charge) when fused or in solution. By doing so, they become capable of conducting electricity.

Electrolytes and electrolyte modifiers include:

- Bicarbonate (HCO_3)
- Calcium ($Ca2+$)
- Magnesium ($Mg2+$)
- Potassium ($K+$)
- Sodium ($Na+$)

Conditions treated with electrolytes and electrolyte modifiers include:

- Hypocalcemia
- Hypokalemia
- Hyponatremia
- Metabolic acidosis
- Prevention and control of seizures

Practice Test 4

Questions

4 - 1

Your postoperative client is to receive potassium chloride. Regarding the administration of intravenous potassium, you know:

1. potassium may be given as a straight intravenous push to avoid fluid overload.
2. potassium is usually mixed 1000 mEq/1000 cc of intravenous fluid.
3. intravenous potassium may only be mixed in normal saline.
4. intravenous potassium should be administered through a large vein.

4 - 2

Furosemide (Lasix) 40 mg is to be administered intravenously to a client with congestive heart failure and excessive weight gain. While the client is receiving Lasix, the nurse will closely observe for:

1. elevated blood pressure.
2. presence of S3 on auscultation of the heart.
3. decrease in serum potassium level.
4. nausea and vomiting.

4 - 3

A client with diabetes is admitted with a urinary tract infection. The initial assessment reveals T-102.5, P-98, BP-97/65, and blood glucose 300 mg/dl. Prescriptions read: Intravenous fluids 5% dextrose in water to infuse at 100 ml/hour, cefoxitin (Mefoxin) 1 gm intravenously every 4 hours, acetaminophen (Tylenol) 650 mg by mouth every 4 hours for temperature greater than 101.5°F or pain, and sliding scale insulin for elevated blood glucose. Which prescriptions will be questioned?

1. cefoxitin (Mefoxin) 1 gm intravenously every 4 hours
2. D5W intravenous infusing 100 ml/h
3. acetaminophen (Tylenol) 650 mg by mouth every 4 hours
4. sliding scale insulin

4 - 4

A client with diabetes is experiencing ketoacidosis and is to receive intravenous fluids containing sodium bicarbonate. Regarding the administration of this intravenous fluid, you know:

1. sodium bicarbonate administration may result in alkalosis.
2. most medications are compatible with sodium bicarbonate.
3. sodium bicarbonate may not be given as an intravenous bolus or push.
4. sodium bicarbonate may only be given intramuscularly.

4 - 5

Your client is to begin a regimen of spironolactone (Aldactone), a potassium-sparing diuretic. You anticipate the following:

1. a sudden drop in serum potassium levels
2. sodium and potassium retention
3. potential lethal cardiac dysrhythmias due to hypokalemia
4. sodium and water excretion, potassium retention

4 - 6

A client presents with a hemoglobin of 19.8 gm/dl. Which of the following medications might have caused this elevation?

1. warfarin (Coumadin)
2. heparin sodium
3. ibuprofen (Motrin)
4. furosemide (Lasix)

4 - 7

A client with a gunshot wound to the abdomen presents at the Emergency Department with a hemoglobin of 7.8 gm/dl. Which of the following do you anticipate administering?

1. packed red blood cells
2. Intralipid
3. hyperalimentation
4. normal saline

4 - 8

A client diagnosed with thrombocytopenia has developed epistaxis, petechiae, and hematuria. Which of the following would be prescribed?

1. Intralipid infusion
2. platelet transfusion
3. furosemide (Lasix) intravenously
4. heparin sodium

4 - 9

A client has developed chronic renal failure and is taking calcium carbonate (Os-Cal). The primary action of calcium carbonate in this situation is to:

1. lower serum phosphate levels.
2. reduce gastric irritation.
3. control blood pressure.
4. regulate bowel function.

4 - 1 0

A client with a history of heart disease complains of shortness of breath. Bilateral crackles are audible and the jugular veins appear distended. Which medication would be most appropriate?

1. furosemide (Lasix)
2. acetylsalicylic acid (aspirin)
3. ampicillin (Unasyn)
4. ranitidine (Zantac)

4 - 1 1

Your client has experienced head injuries. Intracranial pressure is elevated and the heart rate is dropping. Mannitol 1.5 gm/kg of body weight is administered intravenously over 60 minutes as prescribed. You know this medication will:

1. increase the heart rate.
2. lower the blood pressure.
3. act as an antimicrobial.
4. help reduce intracranial pressure.

4 - 1 2

Your client had a thyroidectomy and is receiving thyroid replacement. Serum thyroid studies are within normal limits. However, the client's legs and arms are twitching and the client complains of abdominal cramps. You suggest the following laboratory studies:

1. creatine phosphokinase-MB (CPK-MB)
2. serum calcium
3. serum Dilantin levels
4. comprehensive drug screen

4 - 1 3

Which of the following would be most useful in the prevention of osteoporosis?

1. calcium (Os-Cal)
2. potassium
3. phytonadione (vitamin K_1)
4. ascorbic acid (vitamin C)

4 - 1 4

Your client has developed acute renal failure. Laboratory values indicate: Sodium 155 mEq/l, potassium 5.6 mEq/l, blood urea nitrogen (BUN) 23, and creatinine 2.4. As a consequence of the client's laboratory results, you will anticipate the administration of:

1. Kayexalate.
2. 0.9% sodium chloride solution.
3. diuretics.
4. potassium chloride.

4 - 1 5

A client comes to the Emergency Department after a car accident. Initial vital signs are T-97.4, P-148, BP-86/40, RR-36. The client is cool and clammy. The initial therapy will most likely include:

1. norepinephrine infusion at 5mcg/min.
2. nitroglycerin infusion at 5 mcg/min.
3. normal saline 500 cc intravenous bolus.
4. continue to monitor and record vital signs.

4 - 1 6

In addition to maintaining the body's water, the renal system also balances the electrolyte concentration. Which of the following signs would alert you to an elevation of your client's serum potassium?

1. change in mental status, cardiac arrhythmias, tall and peaked T waves on the electrocardiogram
2. changes in mental status, cardiac arrhythmias, depressed or inverted T waves on the electrocardiogram
3. changes in mental status, muscle weakness or flaccidity
4. cardiac arrhythmias, neuromuscular irritability

4 - 1 7

A young client, determined to lose weight rapidly, has been taking the diuretic furosemide indiscriminately. Which of the following laboratory tests do you anticipate requesting?

1. hemoglobin and hematocrit
2. digoxin level
3. sodium and potassium levels
4. prothrombin time

4 - 1 8

A client's parathyroid glands were removed inadvertently during a thyroidectomy. Which of the following medications do you anticipate administering?

1. potassium chloride
2. glucose
3. calcium gluconate
4. sodium chloride

4-19

Your client has been taking hydro-chlorothiazide (Ezide) for several years and is complaining of anorexia, muscle cramps, and confusion. What is the most likely cause of these symptoms?

1. drug toxicity
2. hyponatremia
3. hypovolemia
4. hypokalemia

4-20

A client is unresponsive and has been brought to the Emergency Department. Initial laboratory results reveal: Serum K+ 3.6 mmol/l, glucose 26 mg/dl, hemoglobin 12.6 gm/dl, carbon dioxide 26.2 mmol/l. You anticipate:

1. dextrose by mouth.
2. 50% dextrose intravenously.
3. 1 unit of packed cells.
4. 10 mEq of KCl over 0.5 hour.

4-21

A client's laboratory work is as follows: Serum glucose 898 mg/dl, arterial blood pH 7.10, HCO_3, 11mEq/l, PCO_2 37 mmHg. You anticipate the need to administer, in addition to insulin, the following treatment:

1. hetastarch 500 intravenously stat
2. immediate intubation and hyperinflation to combat respiratory acidodis
3. 1 unit of packed red blood cells given stat
4. sodium bicarbonate infusion to combat metabolic acidosis

4-22

A client has developed chronic renal failure and is taking aluminum hydroxide (Amphojel). The nurse explains to the client that the primary purpose for this medication in this situation is to:

1. lower serum phosphate levels.
2. reduce gastric irritation.
3. control blood pressure.
4. regulate bowel function.

4 - 2 3

To reduce the risk of cardiac arrhythmias due to transfusions with refrigerated blood, you will:

1. dilute the blood with 0.9% NaCl.
2. warm the blood.
3. rotate the blood gently between your palms.
4. let the blood stand at room temperature for 1 hour.

4 - 2 4

A prescription for cefoxitin (Mefoxin) is to be administered. You know this drug is given for:

1. elevated body temperature.
2. urinary tract infection.
3. elevated blood glucose.
4. pain associated with urination.

4 - 2 5

A client enters the hospital in acute renal failure. The client complains of drowsiness, nausea, and has Kussmaul's breathing. Laboratory tests show a serum potassium of 6.8, serum sodium of 120, and blood pH of 7.2. Which of the following physician's prescriptions should be questioned?

1. polystyrene sodium sulfonate (Kayexalate) 50 gm per rectum as enema
2. 2000-calorie, high-carbohydrate, high-protein diet when nausea subsides
3. hypertonic glucose (25%) 300 cc with regular insulin per intravenous infusion over 1 hour
4. limit po fluids per 8 hours to no more than 100 cc above the urinary output for the previous 8 hours

Practice Test 4

Answers, Rationales, and Explanations

4 - 1

④ **To avoid irritation, a large intravenous bore into a large vein is recommended when administering potassium. Intravenous potassium is very irritating to tissues and veins and may cause irritation at the injection pathway.**

1. Potassium given intravenously must always be diluted. Each dose should be diluted and mixed in 100 to 1000 ml of solution. The mix is usually 40 to 80 mEq/l depending upon the degree of hypokalemia.

2. Potassium given intravenously is usually mixed 40 to 80 mEq/1000 cc, not 1000 mEq/1000 cc.

3. Potassium given intravenously can be mixed with many intravenous solutions, including D5W, normal saline, and Ringer's solution.

Pregnancy Category: C

Client Need: Safe, Effective Care Environment

4 - 2

③ **The nurse will observe for a decrease in serum potassium levels when clients are taking furosemide (Lasix). Normal potassium levels are 3.5 to 5.5 mEq/l. The most significant side effects of Lasix include depletion of potassium (K), sodium (Na), and hypotension. Clients should be specifically monitored for hypokalemia. Furosemide (Lasix) is a loop diuretic that increases excretion of water and electrolytes (e.g., potassium and sodium).**

1. Diuretics tend to lower blood pressure, not elevate it. Therefore, clients receiving loop diuretics should be assessed for hypotension.

2. S3 heart sound is a sign of congestive heart failure, which should improve with the administration of a diuretic like furosemide (Lasix).

4. Lasix may cause nausea and vomiting, but these are mild side effects compared to a decrease in serum potassium levels, which may be life threatening.

Pregnancy Category: C

Client Need: Physiological Integrity

4 - 3

② **The administration of D5W should be questioned in this situation. D5W contains glucose, so it is an inappropriate intravenous solution for a diabetic client. The client's blood glucose is 300 mg/dl. Giving additional glucose would elevate the blood glucose level further. A hypotonic solution of 0.45% sodium chloride (NaCl) is preferred. An intravenous rate of 100 ml/h is appropriate for rehydration.**

1. Cefoxitin (Mefoxin) is the drug of choice for urinary tract infection and would not be questioned.

3. Tylenol can be given as an antipyretic or analgesic and is appropriate for this client's condition.

4. Sliding scale insulin is an appropriate regimen prescribed for short-term management of elevated blood glucose.

Pregnancy Category: C

Client Need: Physiological Integrity

4 - 4

① **Administering sodium bicarbonate may cause alkalosis. Sodium bicarbonate is an electrolyte replenisher and alkalizing agent. Acidotic clients (pH < 7.35) are given sodium bicarbonate to raise the pH. Excessive administration may cause alkalosis (pH > 7.45).**

2. Many medications are incompatible with sodium bicarbonate.

3. Sodium bicarbonate may be given as an intravenous push.

4. Sodium bicarbonate is usually only given by mouth or intravenously.

Pregnancy Category: C

Client Need: Physiological Integrity

4 - 5

④ **You will anticipate sodium and water excretion and potassium retention in clients taking spironolactone (Aldactone). Spironolactone (Aldactone) does not excrete potassium, as do loop diuretics. It is referred to as a potassium-sparing diuretic.**

1. Hypokalemia or a drop in serum potassium levels is not expected with potassium-sparing diuretics such as Aldactone.

2. Sodium and water are excreted, not retained.

3. Cardiac dysrhythmia should not occur because of hypokalemia, since potassium is not excreted.

Pregnancy Category: C

Client Need: Physiological Integrity

4 - 6

④ **Furosemide (Lasix) can produce an elevated hemoglobin. A hemoglobin above 18 gm/dl is referred to as polycythemia (excess of red blood cells). This may be due to an increase in red blood cell production or a decrease in plasma volume, which makes the blood more concentrated with red blood cells. Diuretics such as furosemide (Lasix) can cause such a relative polycythemia by decreasing plasma volume.**

1. Warfarin (Coumadin) is not known to increase red blood cell production or decrease plasma volume. It is an anticoagulant that is used to prevent clot extension or formation.

2. Heparin sodium (an anticoagulant) is not known to increase red blood cell production or decrease plasma volume.

3. Ibuprofen (Motrin) is an anti-inflammatory, antipyretic, and analgesic. It is not known to increase red blood cell production or decrease plasma volume.

Pregnancy Category: C

Client Need: Physiological Integrity

4 - 7

①   **Packed red blood cells are likely to be given in this situation. A normal hemoglobin is between 12 to 16 gm/dl. This client's hemoglobin is extremely low, most likely due to trauma (hemorrhage). The red blood cells need to be replaced.**

2.   Fat emulsion (Intralipid) is a medication administered for the treatment and prevention of essential fatty acid deficiency in clients receiving long-term parenteral nutrition. Intralipids do not elevate hemoglobin levels.

3.   Hyperalimentation refers to intravenous infusions of hypertonic solutions containing enough nutrients to sustain life and maintain a client's growth and development. Hyperalimentation does not directly affect hemoglobin levels.

4.   Normal saline would be helpful as a fluid expander, but this client's hemoglobin indicates a need for packed red blood cells.

Pregnancy Category: NR
Client Need: Health Promotion/Maintenance

4 - 8

②   **Platelet replacement is indicated. Thrombocytopenia (an abnormal decrease in platelet count) may be due to a disease process or drug side effects. Low platelet count (< 20,000/ml) inhibits clot formation and facilitates hemorrhage. Epistaxis (nosebleed), petechiae (small hemorrhagic spots on the skin), and hematuria (blood in the urine) are all signs of this disorder.**

1.   Fat emulsion (Intralipid) infusion is usually a part of parenteral nutrition and is not associated with the treatment of thrombocytopenia.

3.   Furosemide (Lasix) is a loop diuretic given for the treatment of edema associated with congestive heart failure and hepatic and/or renal disease. It does not affect platelet count.

4.   Heparin sodium is an anticoagulant and would be contraindicated in the presence of hemorrhage.

Pregnancy Category: NR
Client Need: Physiological Integrity

4 - 9

①   **Calcium carbonate (Os-Cal) lowers serum phosphate levels. Os-Cal is used in the treatment and prevention of hyperphosphatemia (an excess of phosphates in the blood), a frequent occurrence in end-stage renal disease. Os-Cal binds with phosphates to decrease absorption, thus lowering serum levels.**

2.   Reduction of gastric irritation is not a primary concern for a client with chronic renal failure.

3.   Hypotension is among the side effects of Os-Cal, not the primary action.

4.   Side effects of Os-Cal include: Constipation, nausea, vomiting, and abdominal pain. It is not used to regulate bowel function.

Pregnancy Category: C
Client Need: Physiological Integrity

4 - 1 0

① A prescription for furosemide (Lasix) is appropriate. Furosemide (Lasix) is a loop diuretic whose impact on renal perfusion at the loop of Henle increases urinary output. Shortness of breath, crackles, and jugular vein distention are all cardinal signs of congestive heart failure (accumulation of an abnormal amount of blood in the pulmonary vascular bed). Diuretic therapy is generally indicated. Diuretics decrease circulating volume, which helps in the treatment of congestive heart failure.

2, 3, and 4. Neither aspirin, ampicillin (Unasyn), nor ranitidine (Zantac) has properties that promote diuresis.

Pregnancy Category: C

Client Need: Physiological Integrity

4 - 1 1

④ Mannitol will reduce intracranial pressure. Mannitol is an osmotic diuretic that reduces intracranial pressure by reducing circulating volume.

1. Mannitol is an osmotic diuretic and does not affect heart rate.
2. Mannitol is an osmotic diuretic, and lowering blood pressure would be a side effect.
3. Mannitol is not an antimicrobial medication.

Pregnancy Category: C

Client Need: Physiological Integrity

4 - 1 2

② Serum calcium studies should be suggested. Hypocalcemia is a fairly common consequence of thyroidectomy because the parathyroid glands, which control calcium levels, may be removed accidentally. You would anticipate a prescription for calcium salts.

1. Although one expects an elevated creatine phosphokinase (CPK) level after surgery, there is no indication that the myocardium has been damaged. The MB would indicate myocardium damage.
3. There is no indication that this client is receiving Dilantin.
4. The client has no history of drug abuse. Although some of the client's symptoms may indicate drug withdrawal, the most likely explanation is hypocalcemia.

Pregnancy Category: C

Client Need: Physiological Integrity

4 - 1 3

① Calcium (Os-Cal) is useful in preventing osteoporosis. Osteoporosis is a skeletal disorder characterized by bone mass reduction. One of the major causes of osteoporosis is inadequate calcium intake. Calcium is needed to help form and strengthen bone. Vitamin D promotes the absorption of calcium and phosphorus.

2. Potassium is a mineral and principal cation in intracellular fluid. It aids in regulation of osmotic pressure and acid-base balance. It does not, however, directly affect bone mass.

3. Phytonadione (vitamin K_1) is required for synthesis of blood coagulation factors II, VII, IX, and X but does not affect bone mass.

4. Ascorbic acid (vitamin C) is prescribed in the management of scurvy and some gastrointestinal diseases. Vitamin C does not affect bone mass.

Pregnancy Category: C
Client Need: Health Promotion/Maintenance

4 - 1 4

① You will anticipate the administration of Kayexalate. Kayexalate lowers serum potassium. The normal potassium value is 3.5 to 5.5 mEq/l. A value of 5.6 mEq/l suggests hyperkalemia. Kayexalate is an electrolyte modifier (cation exchange resin) administered to lower serum potassium levels. Each gram of Kayexalate is exchanged for 0.5 to 1 mEq of potassium.

2. Infusing an isotonic solution (0.9%) of sodium chloride would increase sodium retention, which is contraindicated in renal failure.

3. Loop diuretics are the treatment of choice to increase sodium and fluid excretion, but they do not treat hyperkalemia.

4. The client has hyperkalemia. Therefore, potassium is contraindicated.

Pregnancy Category: C
Client Need: Physiological Integrity

4 - 1 5

③ Initial therapy is likely to include normal saline 500 cc intravenous bolus. Fluid resuscitation would be the treatment of choice initially for a trauma client exhibiting signs of shock.

1. A norepinephrine infusion is generally not administered until after a fluid resuscitation attempt.

2. Nitroglycerin is a vasodilator and would lower the blood pressure.

4. The client is exhibiting signs of shock. A replacement fluid such as isotonic (0.9%) normal saline would be an appropriate initial therapy in addition to monitoring and recording vital signs.

Pregnancy Category: NR
Client Need: Physiological Integrity

4 - 1 6

① **Potassium affects the conduction of the myocardium and its contractibility. As a result, markedly elevated serum potassium levels cause arrhythmia (dysrhythmias), electrocardiogram changes (tall T waves), and changes in mental status.**

2. Changes in mental status or cardiac arrhythmias and depressed or inverted T waves on the electrocardiogram are signs of hypokalemia, not hyperkalemia.

3. Changes in mental status or muscle weakness and flaccidity are signs of hypercalcemia, not hyperkalemia.

4. Cardiac arrhythmias (dysrhythmias) and neuromuscular irritability are signs of hypocalcemia and hypokalemia, not hyperkalemia.

Pregnancy Category: C

Client Need: Physiological Integrity

4 - 1 7

③ **A request for sodium and potassium levels will be anticipated. Diuretics promote diuresis (urinary output). In addition to water, urine also contains electrolytes such as sodium and potassium. Persons taking diuretics must be assessed for electrolyte changes that could cause cardiac arrhythmias or central nervous system involvement.**

1. Diuretics such as furosemide do not directly affect hemoglobin and hematocrit.

2. There is no reason to obtain a digoxin level since the client is not taking digoxin.

4. Prothrombin time is obtained when clients are taking the anticoagulant warfarin (Coumadin). There is no evidence that the client is taking any medications other than furosemide.

Pregnancy Category: C

Client Need: Physiological Integrity

4 - 1 8

③ **You will anticipate a prescription for calcium gluconate. The hormone secreted by the parathyroid gland (parathormone) causes calcium to be absorbed from the gastrointestinal tract and from the bone. Because serum levels of calcium are dependent on parathormone's presence, the calcium will need to be replaced.**

1, 2, and 4. Potassium chloride, glucose, and sodium chloride are not directly acted upon by the parathyroid's hormone.

Pregnancy Category: C

Client Need: Physiological Integrity

4 - 1 9

④ **The client's symptoms are characteristic of hypokalemia (potassium depletion). Hydrochlorothiazide (Ezide) is a diuretic (thiazide) that increases excretion of water and sodium by preventing sodium reabsorption in the distal tubules. In addition, excretion of chloride, bicarbonate, magnesium, and potassium takes place. The loss of too much potassium results in hypokalemia and should be treated. Symptoms of hypokalemia include anorexia, muscle cramps, numbness and tingling of lower extremities, confusion, and coma.**

1. Hypotension and tachycardia would suggest drug toxicity.

2. Major symptoms of hyponatremia (sodium depletion) include anxiety, drowsiness and stupor, muscle weakness, convulsions, oliguria, and anuria.

3. Major symptoms of hypovolemia (abnormally decreased volume of circulating fluid) include oliguria, hypotension, and dry skin.

Pregnancy Category: B

Client Need: Physiological Integrity

4 - 2 0

② **You would anticipate the administration of 50% dextrose intravenously. The glucose level is dangerously low and requires immediate attention. Extremely low glucose levels may deprive vital organs of this essential nutrient, even damaging brain cells. A normal serum glucose is 60–115 mg/dl.**

1. No unresponsive person should be given medication by mouth.

3. The client's hemoglobin is not a concern. Normal hemoglobin is 12–14 g/dl in adult females and 14–16 g/dl in adult males.

4. The client's serum potassium is within normal limits (3.5–5.0 mmol/l).

Pregnancy Category: C

Client Need: Physiological Integrity

4 - 2 1

④ **A sodium bicarbonate infusion will treat metabolic acidosis. These laboratory values reveal metabolic acidosis as evidenced by a pH less than 7.35 and an HCO of less than 22 mEq/l. The PCO$_2$ is normal (35–45 mmHg). Sodium bicarbonate is an electrolyte modifier (alkalinizing agent) administered to manage metabolic acidosis.**

1. Hetastarch (Hespan) is a volume expander. There is no evidence that fluid volume replacement is needed.

2. This client's laboratory results are evidence of metabolic, not respiratory, acidosis.

3. There is no indication that the hemoglobin is low.

Pregnancy Category: C

Client Need: Physiological Integrity

4 - 2 2

① **Aluminum hydroxide (Amphojel) lowers serum phosphate levels. Clients in chronic renal failure do not excrete phosphate as they should, and hyperphosphatemia (an excess of phosphates in the blood) may result. Aluminum hydroxide is an antacid electrolyte modifier (hypophosphatemic). It binds with phosphorus in the intestine, and the phosphorous is then excreted via the gastrointestinal tract.**

2. Reducing gastric irritation would not be the primary reason for administering aluminum hydroxide (Amphojel) when a client has chronic renal failure.

3. Aluminum hydroxide (Amphojel) has no affect on blood pressure.

4. Aluminum hydroxide (Amphojel) may affect bowel activity, but its primary action in this situation is the regulation of serum phosphate levels.

Pregnancy Category: NR
Client Need: Physiological Integrity

4 - 2 3

② **To reduce the risk of cardiac arrhythmias due to refrigerated (cold) blood, you will warm the blood.**

1. Diluting blood is not done for the purpose of warming it.

3. Rotating medications such as those in suspension (insulin) helps to resuspend the insulin. Rotating blood, however, is not recommended.

4. Conventional blood warmers should be used to warm blood.

Pregnancy Category: NR
Client Need: Physiological Integrity

4 - 2 4

② **Cefoxitin (Mefoxin) is commonly prescribed for urinary tract infections. It is a broad-spectrum cephalosporin antibiotic. Other usages include treatment of infection in the respiratory tract, on the skin, and in the bones and joints.**

1. Cefoxitin (Mefoxin) is not an antipyretic. It has no effect on body temperature. However, controlling infection may lower the temperature.

3. For immediate management of elevated blood glucose, regular insulin with its rapid onset is the drug of choice, not cefoxitin.

4. Mefoxin is an antibiotic and has no direct effect on pain associated with urination. Dysuria (painful urination) decreases with control of urinary tract infections.

Pregnancy Category: B
Client Need: Health Promotion/Maintenance

4 - 2 5

② **Dietary protein is usually eliminated in acute renal failure to decrease nitrogenous metabolic waste products.**

1. Kayexalate reduces serum potassium by exchanging sodium for potassium ions in the gastrointestinal tract. Inasmuch as this client is hyperkalemic and hyponatremic, this is a reasonable prescription.

3. Hypertonic glucose and insulin promote movement of potassium into the cells, reducing hyperkalemia.

4. Fluid balance must be carefully monitored. Intake should be slightly more than output per 24 hours as rapid changes may occur. Intake is frequently based on the prior 8-hour fluid output.

Pregnancy Category: N/A
Client Need: Health Promotion/Maintenance

Practice Test 5

Gastrointestinal Tract Agents

OVERVIEW

Gastrointestinal tract agents treat, inhibit, and prevent conditions that interfere with the process of digestion: the breakdown, absorption, and elimination of food.

Gastrointestinal tract agents include:

- Adsorbents
- Antacids
- Antidiarrheals
- Antiemetics
- Antiflatulents

- Antiulcer substances
- Digestive enzymes
- Gallstone solubilizers
- Laxatives

ADSORBENTS

Adsorbents easily adhere to other substances. For example, activated charcoal may be administered for its ability to adhere to drugs and poisons and prevent them from being absorbed into the gastrointestinal tract. Adsorbents are generally administered as antagonists (substances that counteract the actions of something else) or antidotes (substances that neutralize poisons or their effects).

Conditions treated with adsorbents include:

- Drug overdoses
- Poisoning

ANTACIDS

Antacids neutralize or reduce acidity in the digestive tract. Antacids elevate gastrointestinal pH, which reduces pepsin effects, which in turn increases esophageal sphincter tone and maintains a strong gastric mucosal barrier.

Conditions treated with antacids include:

- Peptic, duodenal, and gastric ulcers (as adjunctive therapy)
- Esophageal reflux

- Hyperacidity
- Indigestion
- Hyperphosphatemia (for clients in chronic renal failure)

ANTIDIARRHEALS

Antidiarrheals are administered to prevent or treat diarrhea (frequent passage of unformed, watery bowel movements).

Conditions treated with antidiarrheals include:

- Acute nonspecific diarrhea
- Diarrhea associated with carcinoid tumors (tumors located in the intestinal tract, bile ducts, pancreas, bronchus, or ovaries)

- Mild nonspecific diarrhea

ANTIEMETICS

Antiemetics are used to treat or prevent nausea and vomiting. Nausea and vomiting are generally associated with the side effects of drug and radiation therapy as well as some metabolic conditions. Antiemetics inhibit stimulation of the vomiting center in the brain and depress the sensitivity of the vestibular apparatus in the inner ear.

Conditions treated with antiemetics include:

- Motion sickness (prevention and treatment)

- Nausea associated with chemotherapy for cancer (as a preventive)
- Vertigo
- Antiemetics are also used as a preoperative preparation, to prevent nausea or vomiting.

ANTIFLATULENTS

Antiflatulents relieve the painful effects of excess gas in the gastrointestinal tract.

Conditions treated with antiflatulents include:

- Dyspepsia
- Flatulence
- Gastric bloating

ANTIULCER SUBSTANCES

Antiulcer substances are administered to clients who have gastrointestinal ulcers, such as peptic and duodenal ulcers. Antiulcer substances:

- Destroy H. pylori in the gastrointestinal tract
- Inhibit acid secretions
- Neutralize or buffer hydrochloric acid
- Strengthen the mucosal barrier

Conditions treated with antiulcer substances include:

- Duodenal ulcer
- Gastroesophageal reflux
- Heartburn
- Pathologic hypersecretory conditions

DIGESTIVE ENZYMES

Digestive enzymes are normally secreted by the mouth, stomach, and intestines. They are responsible for the decomposition and digestion of food. Enzymes present in digestive juices act upon food to break it down into simpler compounds.

Conditions treated with digestive enzymes include:

- Pancreatic secretion insufficiency
- Steatorrhea (fatty stools as seen in pancreatic diseases)

GALLSTONE SOLUBILIZERS

Gallstone solubilizers dissolve gallstones that are retained in the biliary tract following a cholecystectomy. The most common gallstones are cholesterol-containing stones. Gallstones form when the bile contains more cholesterol than can be maintained in a solution.

Conditions treated with gallstone solubilizers include:

- Gallstones

LAXATIVES

Laxatives are foods or chemicals administered to treat or prevent constipation. The actions of various laxatives are different, but all are administered to relieve constipation.

Laxatives include:

- Bulk-forming substances
- Fecal softeners
- Hyperosmolar substances
- Saline substances
- Stimulants

Conditions treated with laxatives include:

- Chronic constipation
- Laxatives are also used to prepare clients for bowel examination, delivery, and surgery.

Practice Test 5

Questions

5 - 1

Your client is experiencing peptic ulcer disease. Which antiulcer medication has the fewest side effects and least systemic absorption?

1. cimetidine (Tagamet)
2. promethazine (Phenergan)
3. sucralfate (Carafate)
4. ranitidine (Zantac)

5 - 2

A physician has just prescribed prednisone (Orasone) for your client. Which of the following medications is often prescribed to prevent a common side effect of prednisone?

1. potassium chloride, to treat potassium depletion
2. ranitidine (Zantac), to treat peptic ulcer formation
3. nystatin (Mycostatin), to treat secondary infection
4. furosemide (Lasix), to treat sodium retention

5 - 3

A client complaining of "heartburn" asks for an antacid. You will administer:

1. aluminum hydroxide (Amphojel).
2. bisacodyl (Dulcolax).
3. docusate (Colace).
4. ranitidine (Zantac).

5 - 4

Which of the following antacids or antiulcer medications may also be useful in preventing osteoporosis?

1. calcium carbonate (Tums)
2. ranitidine (Zantac)
3. nizatidine (Axid)
4. aluminum hydroxide (Nephrox)

5 - 5

Clients with gastric or duodenal ulcers may be treated with cimetidine (Tagamet), ranitidine (Zantac), or famotidine (Pepcid). Medications such as these promote healing and reduce further ulcer formation by:

1. lowering the pH of gastric secretions, thus reducing tissue irritation.
2. blocking histamine release in the stomach, thus reducing gastric acid production.
3. raising the pH in the stomach and duodenum, thus reducing tissue irritation.
4. coating the stomach and duodenum, thus protecting damaged tissue and allowing it to heal.

5 - 6

Your client was hospitalized after experiencing extensive deep-partial thickness burns. The client has developed Curling's ulcers. You anticipate a prescription for:

1. digoxin (Lanoxin).
2. erythromycin (Erythrocin).
3. ranitidine (Zantac).
4. ganciclovir (Cytovene).

5 - 7

Your client has been taking diphenoxylate/atropine (Lomotil) for diarrhea. Because of the atropine in this medication, you know to assess the client for:

1. bradycardia.
2. tachycardia.
3. excess salivation.
4. urinary incontinence.

5 - 8

Your client had a hemorrhoidectomy. To soften and lubricate the first postoperative bowel movement, you anticipate the administration of mineral oil and a stool softener such as:

1. docusate sodium (Colace).
2. bisacodyl (Dulcolax).
3. calcium polycarbophil (Fiberall).
4. senna (black draught).

5 - 9

Your client has severe gastroesophageal reflux disease. To manage this condition, you anticipate a prescription for ranitidine (Zantac). You know this drug will:

1. decrease gastric acid secretion.
2. increase lower esophageal sphincter pressure.
3. promote gastric emptying.
4. improve peristalsis.

5 - 1 0

Your 18-year-old female client has bulimia nervosa. She is to receive tranylcypromine sulfate (Parnate). You know this medication is administered primarily to:

1. treat underlying anxiety.
2. control frequent weight fluctuations.
3. inhibit the urge to binge.
4. prevent and relieve nausea and vomiting.

5 - 1 1

Your client has ulcerative colitis and is to receive sulfasalazine (Azulfidine). You will teach the client to:

1. take the drug on an empty stomach.
2. avoid exposure to ultraviolet light.
3. observe urine and skin for reddish discoloration.
4. rise slowly from a lying position.

5 - 1 2

A client who has a history of gastric ulcer disease has a sprained ankle and is to receive a medication to relieve pain. For which medication would you anticipate a prescription?

1. ibuprofen
2. acetaminophen
3. aspirin
4. Indocin

5 - 1 3

Following the ingestion of improperly canned tomatoes, your client contracted botulism. You know the treatment of choice for this condition is the administration of:

1. hepatitis A vaccine.
2. the antitoxin.
3. rotavirus vaccine.
4. Crotalidae antivenom.

5 - 1 4

Your client is to receive medication to relieve the symptoms of flatulence and gastric bloating. You will anticipate a prescription for:

1. magnesium oxide.
2. aluminum carbonate.
3. simethicone.
4. calcium carbonate.

5 - 1 5

Your client is experiencing frequent acute diarrhea. For which of the following medications will you anticipate a prescription?

1. dimenhydrinate (Dramamine)
2. metoclopramide (Reglan)
3. lactulose (Cephulac)
4. loperamide (Imodium)

Practice Test 5

Answers, Rationales, and Explanations

5 - 1

③ **Sucralfate (Carafate) will cause the fewest side effects and has the least systemic absorption. Sucralfate (Carafate) is an antiulcer medication that acts as a protective barrier, coating the gastric and duodenal mucosa. Its systemic absorption is low. Clients may take it as a slurry (a thin, watery mixture) usually before meals and at bedtime.**

1. Cimetidine (Tagamet) is systemically absorbed and affects gastric acid secretion by blocking H_2 receptor sites. This medication has many side effects.

2. Promethazine (Phenergan) is an antiemetic, antihistamine, and sedative/hypnotic and is not prescribed for the treatment of peptic ulcers.

4. Ranitidine (Zantac) is systemically absorbed and affects gastric acid secretion by blocking H2 receptor sites. This medication has many side effects.

Pregnancy Category: B

Client Need: Physiological Integrity

5 - 2

② **Ranitidine (Zantac) may be given to prevent the development of peptic ulcer, a common side effect associated with the administration of prednisone.**

1. Prednisone does not cause potassium depletion.

3. Prednisone may suppress the normal immune response, but not just for fungal infections, which is what nystatin treats.

4. Prednisone may cause minimal fluid retention but rarely requires drug intervention. Fluid retention is generally not a concern unless prednisone is administered over a long period in large dosages.

Pregnancy Category: B

Client Need: Health Promotion/Maintenance

5 - 3

① **Aluminum hydroxide (Amphojel) is an antacid that is effective in relieving "heartburn." Aluminum hydroxide acts directly on the stomach's pH, increasing total pH of the stomach.**

2 and 3. Bisacodyl (Dulcolax) and docusate (Colace) are both laxatives.

4. Ranitidine (Zantac) is a histamine H_2 blocker whose overall effect is to increase gastric pH by reducing acid secretion. It is not an antacid.

Pregnancy Category: NR

Client Need: Physiological Integrity

5 - 4

① **Calcium carbonate (Tums) is useful in preventing osteoporosis. Osteoporosis is a skeletal disorder due to a lack of calcium. Tums is a common over-the-counter drug thought to help prevent the development of osteoporosis because it supplies bioavailable calcium.**

2, 3, and 4. Ranitidine (Zantac), nizatidine (Axid), and aluminum hydroxide (Nephrox) do not contain appreciable amounts of bioavailable calcium.

Pregnancy Category: C

Client Need: Health Promotion/Maintenance

5 - 5

② **Cimetidine (Tagamet), ranitidine (Zantac), and famotidine (Pepcid) are all H_2 (histamine) receptor blockers. Histamine, as a vasodilator, dilates vessels in the stomach and increases gastric acid secretion. Blocking histamine production will reduce gastric acid secretion, making the stomach and duodenum less acidic. This allows healing and reduces the likelihood of further tissue damage.**

1. Reducing the pH in the stomach increases its acidity and results in even greater likelihood of tissue damage.

3. Raising the pH in the stomach and duodenum is best accomplished with antacids.

4. Coating the gastric lining and upper intestinal mucosa is accomplished by administering medications like Carafate, an antiulcer agent (protectant). Carafate combines with gastric acid, forming a paste. The ulcer is protected as the paste clings to its surface.

Pregnancy Category: B

Client Need: Physiological Integrity

5 - 6

③ **You will anticipate a prescription for ranitidine (Zantac). Curling's ulcers are duodenal ulcers that may occur in clients who have experienced severe burn trauma. They are not uncommon and are treated with H_2 blockers such as cimetidine and ranitidine.**

1. Digoxin (Lanoxin) is a cardiac glycoside antiarrhythmic and is not used in the treatment of Curling's ulcers.

2. Erythromycin (Erythrocin) is an anti-infective and is not used in the treatment of Curling's ulcers.

4. Ganciclovir (Cytovene) is an antiviral and is not used in the treatment of Curling's ulcers.

Pregnancy Category: C

Client Need: Physiological Integrity

5 - 7

② **Clients receiving high dosages of atropine may experience tachycardia. Atropine is an anticholinergic drug that at low dosages is drying to mucous membranes but at high dosages will block vagal stimulation and increase the heart's rate.**

1. High doses of atropine may cause tachycardia, not bradycardia.

3. Atropine may cause dry mouth, not excessive salivation.

4. Atropine may cause urinary retention, not urinary incontinence.

Pregnancy Category: C

Client Need: Health Promotion/Maintenance

5 - 8

① **Docusate sodium (Colace) is a stool softener (not a stimulant laxative) that softens and lubricates the stool by promoting the incorporation of additional liquid into the stool.**

2 and 4. Bisacodyl (Dulcolax) and senna (black draught) are stimulant laxatives that increase peristalsis by directly affecting the smooth muscle of the intestine. Stimulating laxatives would be excessive following a hemorrhoidectomy.

3. Calcium polycarbophil (Fiberall) is a bulk-forming laxative administered to treat constipation. It would be excessive following a hemorrhoidectomy.

Pregnancy Category: C

Client Need: Health Promotion/Maintenance

5 - 9

① **Ranitidine (Zantac) decreases gastric acid secretion. Ranitidine (Zantac) is an antiulcer agent (a histamine receptor antagonist) that inhibits the action of histamine at the receptor sites and thereby decreases gastric acid secretion.**

2. Ranitidine (Zantac) does not increase lower esophageal sphincter pressure. However, bethanechol (Urecholine) may be prescribed because it has been found to increase lower esophageal sphincter pressure, thereby preventing reflux.

3 and 4. Ranitidine (Zantac) does not promote gastric emptying. However, cisapride (Propulsid) may be prescribed because it promotes gastric emptying, increases lower esophageal sphincter pressure, and improves peristalsis.

Pregnancy Category: B

Client Need: Physiological Integrity

5 - 1 0

③ **Tranylcypromine sulfate (Parnate) is an antidepressant. It is administered to clients experiencing bulimia nervosa to inhibit their urge to binge.**

1. Tranylcypromine sulfate (Parnate) is an antidepressant, not an antianxiety agent.

2. Clients with bulimia have frequent weight fluctuations of 10 pounds or more due to the behaviors of binging and purging. Tranylcypromine sulfate (Parnate) has no effect on this aspect of the condition.

4. Antiemetics prevent and relieve nausea and vomiting; antidepressants do not. Also, clients who self-induce vomiting (purging) do not vomit because they are "sick."

Pregnancy Category: C

Client Need: Physiological Integrity

5 - 1 1

② **Clients should be taught to avoid ultraviolet light since sulfasalazine (Azulfidine) causes photosensitivity. A sunscreen should be used along with protective clothing. Sulfasalazine (Azulfidine) is an uncategorized drug that relieves the symptoms associated with ulcerative colitis and Crohn's disease.**

1. Sulfasalazine (Azulfidine) should be taken with food to decrease gastrointestinal irritation.

3. Clients receiving sulfasalazine (Azulfidine) should be taught that the drug may turn their skin and urine an orange-yellow color, not reddish.

4. Orthostatic hypotension is not associated with the administration of sulfasalazine (Azulfadine). There is no need to warn the client to rise slowly from a lying to a sitting position.

Pregnancy Category: B

Client Need: Health Promotion/Maintenance

5 - 1 2

② **You should anticipate a prescription for acetaminophen (Tylenol) because it is not ulcerogenic (ulcer causing).**

1, 3, and 4. Ibuprofen, aspirin, and Indocin should not be administered to a client with a history of gastric ulcer disease. They are all ulcerogenic (ulcer causing), especially when they are taken in combination.

Pregnancy Category: B

Client Need: Physiological Integrity

5 - 1 3

② **The botulinum antitoxin is the drug of choice for treating the life-threatening condition of botulism. Botulism is a food poisoning associated with the improper canning of certain fruits and vegetables, as well as sausages and smoked and preserved meats and fish. It is caused by the organism Clostridium botulinum.**

1. The hepatitis A vaccine is an active immunization against the hepatitis A virus. A vaccine is not given to treat but to prevent a specific condition. The hepatitis A vaccine has no effect against botulism.

3. The rotavirus vaccine is given to prevent gastroenteritis caused by the rotavirus contained in the offending virus.

4. The Crotalidae antivenom is an anti-snakebite serum obtained from the serum of horses that have been immunized against the venom of several types of pit viper. The Crotalidae antivenom has no effect against the organism that causes botulism.

Pregnancy Category: C

Client Need: Physiological Integrity

5 - 1 4

③ **A prescription for simethicone (Gas-X) would be anticipated. Simethicone is an antiflatulent agent that relieves the symptoms of flatulence (gas) by its defoaming action. Simethicone disperses/prevents the formation of mucus surrounding gas pockets in the gastrointestinal tract.**

1. Magnesium oxide is an antacid and laxative, but it is not an antiflatulent. It is also administered as an oral replacement therapy in the treatment of mild hypomagnesmia.

2. Aluminum carbonate is an antacid. It does not have any antiflatulent effects.

4. Calcium carbonate (Tums) is administered as a calcium supplement and antacid. It does not have antiflatulent effects.

Pregnancy Category: NR

Client Need: Physiological Integrity

5 - 1 5

④ **You will anticipate a prescription for the antidiarrheal drug loperamide (Imodium). This drug is effective in treating diarrhea because it inhibits peristaltic activity.**

1. Dimenhydrate (Dramamine) is an antiemetic administered to treat the symptoms of motion sickness. It does not affect stooling.

2. Metoclopramide (Reglan) is an antiemetic administered to treat the symptoms of nausea and vomiting. It does not affect stooling.

3. Lactulose (Cephulac) is a laxative and would not be administered since it would compound the problem.

Pregnancy Category: B

Client Need: Physiological Integrity

Practice Test 6

Hematologic Agents

OVERVIEW

Hematologic agents are administered as prophylaxis and treatment for various thromboembolytic conditions. They also increase the amount of hemoglobin in the blood, control bleeding, and lyse thrombi.

Hematologic agents include:

- **Anticoagulants**
- **Blood derivatives**
- **Hematinics**
- **Thrombolytic enzymes**

ANTICOAGULANTS

Anticoagulants are used to prevent and treat blood clot (thrombi) extension and formation. Anticoagulants include oral preparations such as warfarin and injectable preparations such as heparin. Anticoagulants do not dissolve blood clots.

Conditions treated with anticoagulants include:

- Cerebral accident
- Bleeding episodes associated with hemophilia
- Malabsorption syndrome
- Pulmonary embolism

BLOOD DERIVATIVES

Blood derivatives are the components (constituents) that make up whole blood.

Blood derivatives include:

- Albumin
- Antihemophilic factor
- Anti-inhibitor coagulant complex
- Factor IX complex
- Factor IX human
- Plasma protein fractions

Conditions treated with blood derivatives include:

- Hemophilia A (Factor VIII deficiency)
- Hemophilia B (Factor IX deficiency)
- Hypovolemic shock

HEMATINICS

Hematinics are drugs or foods used to increase the number of red blood cells, the amount of hemoglobin in the red blood cells, or both.

Conditions treated with hematinics include:

- Megaloblastic anemia
- Pernicious anemia

THROMBOLYTIC ENZYMES

Thrombolytics break down fibrin blood clots by converting plasminogen (a protein found in many body tissues and fluids) to plasmin (fibrolysin). Plasmin then breaks down the fibrin, which lyses (dissolves) blood clots.

Conditions treated with thrombolytic enzymes include:

- Acute myocardial infarction
- Deep vein thrombosis
- Obstructed arteriovenous cannulae
- Pulmonary emboli

Practice Test 6

Questions

6 - 1

An early indicator of warfarin (Coumadin) toxicity is:

1. anemia.
2. hematuria.
3. hypocalcemia.
4. prolonged alopecia.

6 - 2

A client was hospitalized following an ischemic cerebral vascular accident. Prescriptions include: Heparin sodium 1000 units per hour by continuous infusion. Regarding the administration of this drug, you know that:

1. this medication may also be given orally.
2. toxicity of this medication is treated with vitamin K.
3. this medication is a peripheral vasodilator.
4. this medication may cause fatal hemorrhage.

6 - 3

A client comes to the Emergency Department complaining of chest pain. The client has a hemoglobin of 7.5 gm/dl. Which of the following would be administered?

1. norepinephrine (Levophed)
2. oxygen
3. potassium chloride (K-Dur)
4. alprazolam (Xanax)

6 - 4

As you teach your client about oral liquid iron administration, you include instructions to:

1. pour liquid iron into milk prior to drinking.
2. swish and swallow liquid iron preparations.
3. observe for clay-colored stools.
4. use a straw to drink the liquid iron supplement.

6 - 5

A client newly diagnosed with hemophilia A will most likely receive a prescription for which of the following?

1. warfarin (Coumadin)
2. Factor VIII
3. vitamin B_{12}
4. heparin sodium

6 - 6

Which of the following types of medications should be avoided when a client is receiving an anticoagulant?

1. stool softeners
2. antacids
3. salicylates
4. antidepressants

6 - 7

As you prepare to administer an iron preparation, you are aware that iron:

1. may only be given intravenously.
2. may only be given by mouth.
3. injections cause little discomfort.
4. given intramuscularly may stain the skin.

6 - 8

Which of the following do you anticipate administering to a client who experienced a crushed pelvis approximately 1 hour ago?

1. packed red blood cells
2. heparin infusion
3. streptokinase
4. levothyroxine sodium

6 - 9

Ferrous sulfate is prescribed for a 2-year-old with anemia. The nurse teaches the child's mother that the iron will be absorbed better if it is administered with:

1. milk.
2. antacids.
3. antibiotics.
4. vitamin C.

6 - 1 0

A client receiving hemodialysis has a fistula in the forearm. Which of the following is administered to maintain fistula patency?

1. heparin sodium
2. ampicillin sodium (Unasyn)
3. atropine sulfate
4. levothyroxine (Synthroid)

6 - 1 1

Your client was hospitalized following a burn. The client's laboratory results are: Albumin 2.0 gm/dl, potassium 4.5 mEq/l, and chloride 110 mEq/l. For which of the following do you anticipate a prescription?

1. potassium chloride 60 mEq, by mouth, now
2. albumin 25%, 50 ml, now
3. furosemide (Lasix) 80 mg, intravenous, now
4. chloride 0.9%, 1 l, intravenous in one hour

6 - 1 2

Your client is on a daily dosage of warfarin (Coumadin) 5 mg by mouth. Regarding the action of this medication, you know:

1. frequent large portions of leafy green vegetables should be encouraged in the diet.
2. black, tarry-looking stools are an expected effect.
3. a soft toothbrush should be used.
4. this medication is usually taken as needed.

6 - 1 3

A client is experiencing an evolving acute myocardial infarction and is to receive alteplase (t-PA). You know this medication's primary action is to:

1. increase heart rate.
2. elevate blood pressure.
3. lyse blood clots.
4. promote diuresis.

6 - 1 4

You receive a prescription to administer 1 chewable aspirin "stat" for your client. The client is suspected of having an acute myocardial infarction. You know the purpose of this drug in this situation is to:

1. decrease fever.
2. decrease pain in the chest.
3. decrease local discomfort caused by invasive procedures.
4. affect blood clotting.

Practice Test 6

Answers, Rationales, and Explanations

6 - 1

② An early indicator of warfarin (Coumadin) toxicity is hematuria (blood in the urine). Because warfarin (Coumadin) is an anticoagulant, hematuria, as well as large bruises, gastrointestinal bleeding, and bleeding from other body orifices, may indicate toxicity. Clients should be taught to report any symptoms of bleeding or bruising. Clients should also be taught to avoid over-the-counter drugs such as aspirin and ibuprofen, since both potentiate (increase the action of) oral anticoagulants.

1. Anemia is more likely to indicate chronic blood loss or frank hemorrhage and would therefore not be an early indicator of warfarin (Coumadin) toxicity.

3. Administration of warfarin (Coumadin) has no relationship to serum calcium levels such as hypocalcemia.

4. Alopecia (loss of hair) may occur following heparin therapy but not Coumadin therapy.

Pregnancy Category: X

Client Need: Physiological Integrity

6 - 2

④ Heparin sodium may cause fatal hemorrhage. Heparin sodium is an anticoagulant whose inhibition of fibrin formation affects the clotting of blood. Because of this, toxic levels may cause potentially fatal bleeding from nearly any vascular site.

1. Heparin is given only parenterally.

2. Toxic levels of heparin are treated with protamine sulfate. Vitamin K is the antidote for warfarin (Coumadin) overdose.

3. Heparin sodium is not a vasodilatory drug but an anticoagulant.

Pregnancy Category: C

Client Need: Physiological Integrity

6 - 3

② Supplemental oxygen is indicated. Hemoglobin is the iron-containing pigment of the red blood cells. It carries oxygen from the lungs to the tissues. Low hemoglobin levels compromise the body's oxygen transport capacity. A normal hemoglobin is 12–16 gm/dl. A hemoglobin of 7.5 gm/dl is too low.

1. Norepinephrine (Levophed) is a pressor agent (restores blood pressure in acute hypotensive conditions). It does not affect chest pain.

3. Potassium chloride (K-Dur) is an electrolyte and does not affect chest pain.

4. Alprazolam (Xanax) is an antianxiety medication and does not affect chest pain.

Pregnancy Category: NR

Client Need: Physiological Integrity

6 - 4

④ **You will teach clients taking oral iron preparations (Fer-In-Sol syrup) to use a straw. Liquid iron supplements may stain the teeth and gums. A straw is used to avoid teeth and gum contact with the liquid iron.**

1. Concurrent milk consumption may decrease iron absorption. Therefore, it is not recommended that oral iron preparations be taken with milk.
2. To swish and then swallow oral liquid iron preparation may stain the teeth and gums.
3 Iron supplements may darken the stool, not cause them to be clay colored.

Pregnancy Category: A
Client Need: Health Promotion/Maintenance

6 - 5

② **Factor VIII is the most likely prescription for the treatment of hemophilia A. Hemophilia A is a hereditary bleeding disorder characterized by a deficiency of clotting factors. Factor VIII is the most common deficiency and replacement of it is the treatment.**

1. Warfarin (Coumadin) is an anticoagulant and would increase the tendency to bleed.
3. Vitamin B_{12} is not deficient in clients with hemophilia A. It is, however, prescribed to treat pernicious anemia.
4. Heparin sodium is an anticoagulant and would increase the tendency to bleed.

Pregnancy Category: C
Client Need: Physiological Integrity

6 - 6

③ **Salicylates should be avoided when anticoagulant therapy is administered. Salicylates such as aspirin (acetylsalicylic acid) block or impede the production of prostaglandin (an unsaturated fatty acid) that helps to form blood clots. Salicylates may cause bleeding in persons already taking an anticoagulant such as heparin or warfarin.**

1, 2, and 4. There is no indication that stool softeners, antacids, or antidepressants should be avoided because of anticoagulant therapy.

Pregnancy Category: C
Client Need: Safe, Effective Care Environment

6 - 7

④ **Intramuscular injections of iron may stain the skin. Iron may be given intramuscularly in the form of iron dextran for those who are unable to swallow or absorb oral dosages. Because intramuscular injections of iron may cause staining of the skin, it is best to use the Z-track method so that the iron does not come to the skin's surface.**

1 and 2. Iron may be given by mouth, intramuscularly, or intravenously.

3.   Injections of iron are painful.

Pregnancy Category: C
Client Need: Safe, Effective Care Environment

6 - 8

① **Packed red blood cells may be given when large bones, such as the pelvis, are crushed. Bone is very vascular. Crushing a large bone often causes the client to lose circulating blood by internal hemorrhage. Replacement of circulating volume is essential to ensure that tissue perfusion will not be compromised.**

2.   Heparin is an anticoagulant and would increase bleeding.

3.   Streptokinase is an antithrombolytic that would facilitate bleeding.

4.   Levothyroxine is a thyroid hormone and has no impact on circulating blood volume.

Pregnancy Category: NR
Client Need: Health Promotion/Maintenance

6 - 9

④ **Vitamin C increases the absorption of iron if taken concurrently. Milk, antacids, and most antibiotics can interfere with the absorption of iron if taken at the same time. It might be recommended that the child take the iron preparation with orange juice.**

1, 2, and 3. Milk, antacids, and antibiotics will interfere with the absorption of iron if taken concurrently.

Pregnancy Category: NR
Client Need: Health Promotion/Maintenance

6 - 1 0

① **Heparin sodium is an anticoagulant whose impact on fibrin formation helps prevent blood from clotting. Heparin is used during hemodialysis to prevent blood clots from forming, which in turn, prevents peripheral ischemia and strokes.**

2. Ampicillin sodium (Unasyn) is an anti-infective that kills bacteria by binding to their cell walls. It is not an anticoagulant and therefore does not affect patency of fistulas.

3. Atropine sulfate is an antiarrhythmic and anticholinergic used to treat bradycardia and decrease secretions preoperatively. It does not affect patency of fistulas.

4. Levothyroxine (Synthroid) is a synthetic hormone used to manage hypothyroidism by increasing the metabolic rate of body tissues. It does not affect patency of fistulas.

Pregnancy Category: C

Client Need: Health Promotion/Maintenance

6 - 1 1

② **A prescription for albumin is anticipated. Albumin is a protein essential in regulating the exchange of water between plasma and the spaces between cells (interstitial compartment). The normal range of albumin is 3.2 to 4.5 gm/dl. Because the client's albumin is markedly low, a replacement would be indicated.**

1. The potassium is within the normal range of 3.5 to 5.5 mEq/l.

3. Furosemide (Lasix) is a diuretic. There is no indication that a diuretic is necessary.

4. The chloride is within the normal range of 90 to 110 mEq/l.

Pregnancy Category: C

Client Need: Physiological Integrity

6 - 1 2

③ **Clients receiving warfarin sodium (Coumadin) should use soft toothbrushes. Warfarin (Coumadin) is an oral anticoagulant that affects the formation of clotting factors. Caution should be taken during its administration to prevent bruising, bleeding, or any skin or mucous membrane tears, since hemorrhage may result.**

1. Leafy green vegetables are discouraged because they contain vitamin K, which counteracts the action of warfarin (Coumadin).

2. The presence of black, tarry-looking stools could indicate gastrointestinal bleeding, which is a reportable condition associated with Coumadin overdosage.

4. Warfarin (Coumadin) is taken daily, at the same time each day.

Pregnancy Category: X

Client Need: Health Promotion/Maintenance

6 - 1 3

③ **Alteplase (t-PA) lyses blood clots. Thrombolytic medications (agents that dissolve thrombi) such as alteplase (t-PA) cause fibrinolysis. Thrombolytics activate plasminogen by converting it to plasmin. The plasmin in turn lyses fibrin clots.**

1, 2, and 4. Any change in heart rate, blood pressure, and diuresis would be a result of changes in cardiac output as a consequence of the success of fibrinolysis.

Pregnancy Category: C
Client Need: Physiological Integrity

6 - 1 4

④ **Aspirin acts against platelet aggregation and impedes blood clotting. Aspirin administration during the acute management of a myocardial infarction may decrease mortality. Aspirin is a nonopioid analgesic, nonsteroidal anti-inflammatory, antipyretic, antiplatelet medication.**

1. Although aspirin is an antipyretic, it would not be given for this reason in this client's situation.

2. Aspirin is an analgesic. However, in this situation it would not be given for its analgesic properties.

3. There is no indication that the client is having an invasive procedure.

Pregnancy Category: D
Client Need: Physiological Integrity

Practice Test 7

Hormonal Agents

OVERVIEW

Hormonal agents treat, prevent, and inhibit conditions that interfere with the function of the endocrine glands, the hormones they secrete, and the organs they innervate.

Hormonal agents include:

- Androgens and anabolic steroids
- Antidiabetic agents and glucagon
- Corticosteroids
- Estrogens and progestins
- Gonadotropins
- Parathyroid-like substances
- Pituitary hormones
- Thyroid hormones and thyroid hormone antagonists

ANDROGENS AND ANABOLIC STEROIDS

ANDROGENS promote masculinization. The male hormones, testerone and its derivatives, are known as androgens and are secreted under the influence of the pituitary gland. Androgens aid in the development and maintenance of male sex characteristics. Androgens also facilitate the tissue-building process.

Conditions treated with androgens include:

- Delayed puberty
- Hypogonadism (abnormally decreased gonadal function)

ANABOLIC STEROIDS are synthetic drugs chemically related to androgens. They promote tissue processes.

Conditions treated with anabolic steroids include:

- Metastatic breast cancer in women
- Postmenopausal and senile osteoporosis

ANTIDIABETIC AGENTS AND GLUCAGON

Antidiabetic agents and glucagons (a polypeptide hormone that increases blood glucose) are administered to treat diabetes mellitus. The six major categories of antidiabetics are:

(1) Insulin

(2) Sulfonylureas

(3) Alpha-glucosidase inhibitors

(4) Biquanides

(5) Thiazolinediones

(6) Meglitinide insulin

(1) Insulin

Insulin is a protein normally secreted by the beta cells of the isles of Langerhans in the pancreas. Insulin is essential for the correct metabolism of blood glucose and for proper maintenance of blood glucose levels. Without the right secretions of insulin, carbohydrates and fats are not properly metabolized and hyperglycemia and glycosuria occur.

Conditions treated with insulin include:

- Diabetes mellitus
- Diabetic ketoacidosis

(2) Sulfonylureas

Sulfonylureas are oral hypoglycemic agents used to control blood glucose in adult-onset noninsulin-dependent diabetes mellitus (NIDDM), when diet alone is not adequate.

Conditions treated with sulfonylureas include:

- Type 2 noninsulin-dependent diabetes mellitus (NIDDM)

(3) Alpha-Glucosidase Inhibitors

Alpha-glucosidase inhibitors influence the activity of enzymes involved in the metabolism of carbohydrates. As a result, blood sugar levels rise more gradually and sudden increases and decreases are avoided.

Conditions treated with alpha-glucosidase inhibitors include:

- Type 2 noninsulin-dependent diabetes mellitus (NIDDM)

(4) Biquanides

Biquanides help decrease blood sugar levels by decreasing productivity of glucose in the liver. Biquanides also prevent weight loss at the onset of use and help normalize blood fat and cholesterol levels.

Conditions treated with biquanides include:

- Type 2 noninsulin-dependent diabetes mellitus (NIDDM)

(5) Thiazolinediones

Thiazolinediones help reduce insulin resistance (help increase insulin sensitivity).

Conditions treated with thiazolinediones include:

- Type 2 noninsulin-dependent diabetes mellitus (NIDDM)

(6) Meglitinide Insulin

Meglitinide is another insulin designed to treat postprandial (after a meal) hyperglycemia. It increases insulin release more quickly than the sulfonylureas. It is glucose-dependent and decreases as the client's blood glucose level drops. Because of its short half-life, the potential for accumulation is minimal.

Conditions treated with meglitinide include:

- Type 2 noninsulin-dependent diabetes mellitus (NIDDM)

CORTICOSTEROIDS

Corticosteroids are hormones (steroids) secreted directly into the bloodstream by the adrenal cortex (outer portion of the adrenal glands). There are three types of these steroid hormones: glucocorticoids, mineralocorticoids, and androgens. GLUCOCORTICOIDS influence the metabolism of sugars, fats, and proteins within body cells and also have a potent anti-inflammatory effect. MINERALOCORTICOIDS regulate mineral salts (electrolytes). Maintaining a normal balance of salts and water in the tissues and blood is essential for a healthy, functioning body. ANDROGENS are male and female hormones that maintain secondary sex characters. (These hormones are also produced in the ovaries and the testes.)

Conditions treated with corticosteroids include:

- Addison's disease
- Adrenal insufficiency
- Feminization
  (female secondary characteristics in a man)
- Hypopituitarism
- Rheumatoid arthritis
- Virilism
  (male secondary sex characteristics in a woman)

ESTROGENS AND PROGESTINS

The estrogens and progestins (progesterone) are the two endogenous female hormones. They are secreted under the influence of the anterior pituitary gland. The three estrogenic hormones are known as estradiol, estrone, and estriol. The ESTROGENS develop and maintain the female reproductive system as well as the primary and secondary sex characteristics. PROGESTIN (progesterone) is responsible for changes in the uterine endometrium, the preparation for implantation of the blastocyst, development of the maternal placenta, and development of the mammary glands.

Conditions treated with estrogens and progestins include:

- Abnormal uterine bleeding
- Prostate cancer
- Primary ovarian failure

GONADOTROPINS

Gonads are the embryonic sex glands before differentiation into the male testis or the female ovary. Follicle-stimulating hormones (FSH) and luteinizing hormones (LH) are known as gonadotropins because they influence the organs of reproduction (the gonads) in both sexes. In males and females, FSH and LH influence the secretion of sex hormones, the development of secondary sex characteristics, and the reproductive cycle.

Conditions treated with gonadotropins include:

- Failure to produce ova and/or failure to ovulate
- Failure of the testes to descend
- Failure to produce sperm

PARATHYROID-LIKE SUBSTANCES

The parathyroid gland consists of four small endocrine glands found on the posterior side of the thyroid. Overactivity (hyperparathyroidism) and underactivity (hypoparathyroidism) are the usual causes for the various conditions associated with the parathyroid gland.

Conditions treated with parathyroid-like substances include:

- Hyperparathyroidism
- Hypoparathyroidism
- Kidney stones (hypercalcemia)
- Hypocalcemia (tetany)
- Paget's disease (osteitis deformans)
- Hypocalcemia in clients on chronic dialysis

PITUITARY HORMONES

The pituitary is a pea-sized gland found at the base of the brain in a small pocket-like cavity called the sella turcica. There are two lobes of the pituitary gland, the anterior lobe (adenohypophysis) and the posterior lobe (neurohypophysis).

The ANTERIOR PITUITARY secretes hormones that influence the growth of bone tissue, the thyroid gland and its secretions, the adrenal cortex and its secretions, and the secretion of hormones associated with the ovaries in females and the testes in males.

The POSTERIOR PITUITARY secretes hormones that influence the reabsorption of water by the kidney tubules, increase the blood pressure by constricting arterioles, maintain labor during childbirth, and cause production of milk from the mammary glands.

Conditions treated with pituitary hormones include:

- Growth failure in children
- Temporary polyuria and polydipsia associated with pituitary trauma

THYROID HORMONES AND THYROID HORMONE ANTAGONISTS

Natural thyroid hormones are secreted directly into the bloodstream by the thyroid gland, located in the neck, anterior to and partially surrounding the thyroid cartilage and upper rings of the trachea. Underactivity (hypothyroidism) and overactivity (hyperthyroidism) are the usual causes for the various conditions associated with the thyroid gland. Synthetic thyroid hormone medications may be administered to treat conditions of the thyroid gland.

HYPOTHYROIDISM is caused by a deficiency of thyroid hormones, resulting in an abnormally slow body metabolism.

Medications used to treat hypothyroidism include:

- Liothyronine sodium (Cytomel)
- Liotrix (Euthroid)

Conditions treated with thyroid hormones include:

- Congenital hypothyroidism
- Cretinism
- Hypothyroidism
- Myxedema
- Nontoxic goiter

HYPERTHYROIDISM is the condition caused by an excessive secretion of thyroid hormones, which results in an abnormally accelerated basal metabolic rate. THYROID HORMONE antagonists are drugs that counteract the action of the thyroid hormones.

Thyroid hormone antagonists used to treat hyperthyroidism include:

- Methimazole (Tapazole)
- Potassium iodine, saturated solution (SSKI)
- Radioactive iodine (sodium iodide) 131

Conditions treated with thyroid hormone antagonists include:

- Hyperthyroidism
- Thyroid cancer
- Thyrotoxic crisis
- Thyroid hormone antagonists are also used to prepare clients for thyroidectomy.

Practice Test 7

Questions

7 - 1

A client is taking 0.1 mg of levothyroxine (Synthroid) per day. What teaching does the client need in relation to this medication?

1. Take medication with meals.
2. Do not substitute generic brands.
3. Dosages can be self-adjusted based on energy needs.
4. Expect to lose 10 to 15 pounds within the first 6 months.

7 - 2

A client experiencing diabetic ketoacidosis is to receive 10 units per hour of a regular insulin infusion. The pharmacy dispensed a bag that contains 100 units of insulin in 250 cc of fluid. At what rate will you deliver this infusion?

1. 2.5 cc per hour
2. 10 cc per hour
3. 25 cc per hour
4. 100 cc per hour

7 - 3

Which of the following might be indicated for a 58-year-old female developing osteoporosis?

1. glucocorticoid therapy
2. heparin therapy
3. vitamin C replacement
4. estrogen replacement

7 - 4

A client with Type 2 diabetes is experiencing elevated blood glucose levels, which are being controlled with sliding scale insulin. When using a sliding scale to control blood glucose, the nurse will administer:

1. 70/30 insulin.
2. Regular insulin.
3. NPH insulin.
4. PZI insulin.

7 - 5

A client is to receive 12 units of Regular insulin and 26 units of NPH insulin subcutaneously daily. Which procedure is correct?

1. Store all insulin in the refrigerator.
2. Massage the injection site after administration.
3. Draw up the NPH insulin first and then the Regular insulin.
4. Roll the NPH insulin bottle between the palms of the hands prior to drawing it up.

7 - 6

Your client will be discharged with a prescription for levothyroxine (Synthroid) 0.1 mg by mouth daily. Included in your discharge teaching are the following instructions:

1. Take this medication only as needed.
2. Take this medication at hour of sleep.
3. Take this medication daily in the a.m.
4. Expect palpitations of the heart.

7 - 7

The nurse understands that clients receiving oral hypoglycemic agents (OHAs) like glyburide (Glynase Pres Tab):

1. do not need to maintain a regular schedule of meals and activity.
2. are likely to maintain normal blood glucose levels.
3. should discontinue use if pregnant or breastfeeding.
4. may become allergic to insulin.

7 - 8

A 22-year-old client is admitted to your department with a blood glucose of 822 mg/dl and an arterial blood pH of 7.02. The client is in diabetic ketoacidosis and is unresponsive. The insulin type and route you anticipate administering is:

1. Humulin N given intravenously.
2. Humulin R given intravenously.
3. Humulin 70/30 given intravenously.
4. Humulin N given subcutaneously only.

7 - 9

Your client has a head injury and is to be given dexamethasone (Decadron) 10 mg intravenously stat. You know the purpose of this medication is to:

1. decrease bleeding.
2. sedate the client.
3. decrease inflammation.
4. provide pain relief.

7 - 1 0

A client with diabetes has been taking glipizide (Glucotrol) 5 mg by mouth daily for the past 4.5 years. Blood glucose levels have been well controlled. After a recent myocardial infarction, the client began taking metoprolol (Lopressor) 50 mg twice daily by mouth. You anticipate:

1. increasing glipizide (Glucotrol) to 10 mg.
2. no change in medications.
3. decreasing glipizide (Glucotrol) to 2.5 mg daily.
4. discontinuing glipizide (Glucotrol).

7 - 1 1

Your client has been controlling elevated glucose levels with a dietary regimen. The client has just begun receiving prednisone (Orasone) for the treatment of lymphoma. The serum glucose is elevated. You attribute this to:

1. an unrelated worsening of the diabetes mellitus.
2. a laboratory error, since prednisone tends to lower serum glucose levels.
3. permanent pancreatic damage due to prednisone therapy.
4. a side effect of corticosteroid therapy that is generally reversible.

7 - 1 2

Your postoperative client is receiving tamoxifen (Nolvadex) 20 mg twice a day by mouth as adjunct therapy for breast cancer. When the client asks about the purpose of this drug, your best response will be:

1. "This drug will destroy any cancer cells that may have escaped into your system when you had surgery."
2. "This medication prevents your body from producing estrogen, which could stimulate the growth of any remaining tumor cells."
3. "This medication will stimulate your body's own immune system to produce substances that seek out and destroy abnormal cells."
4. "This drug causes more calcium to become deposited in your bones, which helps to prevent the spread of cancer."

7 - 1 3

Your client is taking insulin lispro injections (Humalog) for the treatment of Type 2 diabetes. You will teach the client that the onset of this insulin is from:

1. 0.3 h to 0.5 h.
2. 1 h to 2 h.
3. 2 h to 4 h.
4. 4 h to 6 h.

7 - 1 4

NPH insulin 20 units and regular insulin 6 units have been prescribed for your client every morning. The client is on a sliding scale dosage for coverage of blood sugar patterns. The client's 7 a.m. blood sugar was 200 mg/dl. This blood sugar level requires coverage with 6 units of Regular insulin. The appropriate insulin dosage for this client at this time is:

1. 20 units of NPH; 6 units of Regular.
2. 20 units of NPH; 12 units of Regular.
3. 26 units of NPH; 6 units of Regular.
4. 26 units of NPH; 12 units of Regular.

7 - 1 5

Your client has no medical history other than arthritis, for which a glucocorticoid has been prescribed. The client's serum glucose today is 210 mg/dl. You understand that:

1. the glucocorticoid medication has caused this precipitous drop in blood sugar.
2. glucocorticoids stimulate the release of glucagon.
3. glucocorticoids have damaged the pancreas.
4. serum glucose is elevated due to the glucocorticoid effect on carbohydrate metabolism.

7 - 1 6

Your client is to receive a 7:00 a.m. dosage of NPH insulin before breakfast. The most likely time for a hypoglycemic reaction is:

1. during the early morning hours.
2. within 4 hours of administration.
3. between the noon and evening meals.
4. before bedtime.

7 - 1 7

Your client has been diagnosed with diabetes insipidus. In addition to accurate fluid management and assessment of daily weight, you anticipate the administration of:

1. glipizide 10 mg intravenously, daily.
2. glipizide 10 mg by mouth, daily.
3. vasopressin 10 units intravenously, daily.
4. vasopressin 10 units subcutaneously, daily.

7 - 1 8

As you prepare to administer your client's dosage of levothyroxine (Synthroid), you notice that the client's heart rate is 146 beats per minute. You will:

1. administer the medication as prescribed.
2. begin cardiopulmonary resuscitation.
3. withhold the dosage and notify the physician.
4. anticipate a dosage increase.

7 - 1 9

A client hospitalized for an acute exacerbation of multiple sclerosis is to be discharged on prednisone. The client has been instructed to continue taking the medication for 4 weeks. What is essential for the client to know about prednisone?

1. The dosage of prednisone should be tapered off gradually.
2. The client is to take the same dosage each day until the prescription is finished.
3. The drug should be taken before meals on an empty stomach.
4. The client will need to increase salt intake to prevent sodium depletion.

7 - 2 0

A 60-year-old female client is to receive the calcium supplement calcitonin-salmon (Calcimar) and estrogen replacement therapy for prevention of osteoporosis. The client has also been instructed to walk 1 to 2 miles daily. This treatment is designed to:

1. reduce calcium resorption and increase calcium laydown in the bones.
2. reduce the vasomotor instability associated with menopause.
3. prevent osteoporosis.
4. prevent the formation of blood clots.

7 - 2 1

You have just administered glucagon intra-venously. You know that an important nursing action associated with the administration of this drug is to:

1. anticipate giving a stat dosage of intra-venous insulin.
2. implement nothing by mouth (NPO) for at least 12 hours.
3. anticipate the administration of sodium bicarbonate intravenously stat.
4. encourage carbohydrates by mouth.

7 - 2 2

You know that glucagon is given to combat insulin shock. You also know that a secondary action of this medication is to:

1. decrease the heart rate.
2. increase the heart rate.
3. manage hypertensive crisis.
4. act as an antiviral agent.

7 - 2 3

During the admission assessment, your client says, "I take insulin" and refers to it as "the long-acting kind." You know that this:

1. is the same as NPH.
2. is now obsolete.
3. lasts up to 8 hours.
4. lasts up to 36 hours.

7 - 2 4

A client is admitted with acute appendicitis. The client is to receive nothing by mouth. The client says, "I am supposed to take glyburide (DiaBeta) 5 mg by mouth daily." The client's glucose level on admission is 362 mg/dl. You are to administer: 10 units Humulin R subcutaneously, now. You explain to your client that the reason for this injection is:

1. the glyburide is not effective.
2. the oral medication plus subcutaneous insulin are needed.
3. subcutaneous insulin is only temporary while the client is NPO.
4. an adjustment needs to be made because the elevation in blood glucose is inexplicable.

7 - 2 5

Your client has Cushing's syndrome and has developed ulcerative colitis. Today's medication prescriptions include: Prednisolone (Predsol) retention enema, 20 mg at hour of sleep every night for 2 weeks. You will:

1. teach the client how to self-administer these enemas, which are to be retained for 30 minutes.
2. withhold the enema and consult with the physician.
3. give the enema as prescribed since it has no systemic effects.
4. anticipate a prescription for a less irritating enema, such as bisacodyl.

7 - 2 6

Which one of the following sulfonylureas should not be administered to treat an alcoholic's Type 2 diabetes?

1. chlorpropamide
2. tolazamide
3. repaglinide
4. glimepiride

7 - 2 7

You are teaching your diabetic client about the insulin lispro (Humalog). You will teach the client that this insulin:

1. has an onset of less than 30 minutes.
2. peaks between 2 to 4 hours.
3. lasts 5 to 7 hours.
4. should be taken 20 to 30 minutes before meals.

7 - 2 8

A client is receiving the thyroid hormone replacement levothyroxine and has been scheduled for an I 131 Uptake study. You know the client must discontinue the levothyroxine:

1. 2 weeks before the study.
2. 3 weeks before the study.
3. 4 weeks before the study.
4. 5 weeks before the study.

Practice Test 7

Answers, Rationales, and Explanations

7 - 1

② **No substitute generic brands of levothyroxine (Synthroid) should be taken since preparations may vary. It is important that consistent and appropriate thyroid levels be maintained. Morning dosage is recommended to prevent insomnia.**

1. Synthroid does not have to be taken with meals. It is, however, recommended that it be taken at the same time each day to establish consistency.

3. The dosage of Synthroid should not be self-adjusted. Dosages should be adjusted based on serum laboratory values and under the direction of a physician.

4. Clients taking Synthroid may experience weight loss as a result of increased basal metabolic rate, but weight loss may not occur in all clients.

Pregnancy Category: A
Client Need: Health Promotion/Maintenance

7 - 2

③ **25 cc per hour will be delivered:**

100 units : 250 cc :: 10 units : X

100X = 2500

X = 25 cc

1, 2, and 4 are incorrect rates per hour.

Pregnancy Category: NR
Client Need: Physiological Integrity

7 - 3

④ **Estrogen replacement is indicated for menopausal women who are developing osteoporosis. Osteoporosis is a disease of the bone characterized by reduction of bone mass. It may be seen in elderly men and women, but it advances more rapidly in women following menopause because the drop in estrogen levels at menopause causes accelerated bone resorption (bone loss). In menopausal women, estrogen replacement decreases the rate of bone resorption and has been found to aid in the treatment of osteoporosis.**

1 and 2. Glucocorticoid and heparin therapies have an adverse effect on clients with osteoporosis because both affect calcium use.

3. Vitamin C does not play a large role in bone formation. However, vitamin D does help in the absorption of calcium and is used in the treatment of osteoporosis.

Pregnancy Category: X
Client Need: Health Promotion/Maintenance

7 - 4

② **Regular insulin administered subcutaneously should be given when insulin is given based on a sliding scale. Regular insulin is always used because of its rapid onset and short duration of action. The onset of subcutaneous Regular insulin is 13 to 60 minutes, peak 2 to 4 hours, duration 5 to 7 hours.**

1. 70/30 is a premixed dose of NPH (intermediate-acting insulin) and Regular (rapid-acting insulin). This combination is undesirable for short-term management of hyperglycemia because of the intermediate-acting insulin. The onset of intermediate-acting insulin is 1 to 4 hours, peak is 6 to 12 hours, and duration 18 to 28 hours.

3. Due to its delayed onset and prolonged duration of action, NPH insulin is not suitable for short-term treatment of elevated blood sugar.

4. PZI is a long-acting insulin. Only short-acting insulin (Regular) should be used in a sliding scale insulin regimen. Regular insulin will rapidly lower elevated blood glucose.

Pregnancy Category: NR

Client Need: Physiological Integrity

7 - 5

④ **NPH insulin is an intermediate-acting insulin. Since NPH insulin is in suspension, it should be rolled between the palms of the hands to thoroughly mix prior to withdrawing the dosage. Shaking NPH insulin can cause an inaccurate dose to be administered.**

1. Insulin may be left at room temperature for up to 4 weeks unless the room temperature is higher than 85° Fahrenheit or below freezing.

2. After injecting insulin, some pressure should be applied to the site while the needle is being withdrawn and the swab should be held in place for a few seconds. The site should not be massaged, as this causes bleeding and tissue irritation.

3. When mixing an intermediate-acting insulin with Regular insulin, the Regular insulin should always be drawn up first due to chemical reactions that interfere with the effectiveness of the insulin. Remember, clear to cloudy.

Pregnancy Category: NR

Client Need: Health Promotion/Maintenance

7 - 6

③ **Levothyroxine (Synthroid) is a synthetic hormone and is usually taken daily upon arising to avoid potential insomnia and to maintain appropriate serum levels.**

1. Levothyroxine (Synthroid) should be taken daily in the a.m. on schedule to maintain appropriate serum levels. It is not to be taken as needed.

2. It is preferable to take levothyroxine (Synthroid) upon arising to avoid insomnia, not at hour of sleep.

4. Palpitations and chest pain are reportable conditions that may indicate levothyroxine (Synthroid) toxicity.

Pregnancy Category: A

Client Need: Physiological Integrity

7 - 7

③ **Oral hypoglycemic agents (OHAs) such as glyburide (Glynase Pres Tabs) are contraindicated in pregnant and breastfeeding women because they cross the placenta barrier and are excreted in milk.**

1. Regular meals, activity, and rest are very important for clients taking oral hypoglycemics.
2. Blood sugar levels may not remain within normal limits while clients are on oral hypoglycemics. Clients need to know the signs of both hypoglycemia and hyperglycemia.
4. Oral hypoglycemics are not an insulin substitute and do not have any association with possible allergy to insulin. They stimulate insulin production and cellular insulin receptors.

Pregnancy Category: B
Client Need: Health Promotion/Maintenance

7 - 8

② **Humulin R will be administered intravenously. This client is experiencing diabetic ketoacidosis. A rapid-acting insulin such as Humulin R is given intravenously and is appropriate for the treatment of ketoacidosis. Humulin R insulin has an onset between 10 to 30 minutes, peak action between 15 to 30 minutes, and a duration between 30 to 60 minutes. Regular insulin is the only insulin that can be administered intravenously. The normal pH is 7.35 to 7.45. The normal blood glucose is 60 to 115 mg/100 ml of blood.**

1. Humulin N may not be given intravenously.
3. Humulin 70/30 may not be given intravenously.
4. Humulin N is given subcutaneously and would not take effect until 1 to 3 hours after administration, which is inappropriate when treating ketoacidosis.

Pregnancy Category: NR
Client Need: Physiological Integrity

7 - 9

③ **Dexamethasone (Decadron) decreases inflammation. Dexamethasone is a glucocorticoid anti-inflammatory agent and affects inflammation by altering prostaglandin synthesis.**

1. Dexamethasone may increase, not decrease, prothrombin time. Guaiac-positive stools should be reported.
2. Dexamethasone is not a sedative/hypnotic.
4. Dexamethasone is not an analgesic.

Pregnancy Category: C
Client Need: Physiological Integrity

7 - 1 0

③ **Glipizide (Glucotrol) should be decreased to 2.5 mg because it has a tendency to increase hypoglycemia when taken with a beta-adrenergic blocker like Lopressor.**

1. A combination of glipizide 10 mg and metoprolol (Lopressor) 50 mg would cause a decrease in serum glucose.
2. Unless there is a decrease in the glipizide, there will be a decrease in the serum glucose.
4. Glipizide and metoprolol (Lopressor) may be taken concurrently with careful monitoring of blood glucose levels.

Pregnancy Category: C
Client Need: Physiological Integrity

7 - 1 1

④ **You attribute the elevation of serum glucose to a side effect of corticosteroid therapy that is generally reversible. Glucocorticoids affect the conversion of fats and carbohydrates to glucose, which tends to elevate serum glucose levels.**

1. There is no reason to think that the diabetes is worse. What we do know is that prednisone tends to elevate serum glucose levels.
2. Prednisone tends to elevate serum glucose levels, not lower them.
3. There is no indication of permanent pancreatic injury due to the corticosteroid therapy.

Pregnancy Category: NR
Client Need: Physiological Integrity

7 - 1 2

② **Tamoxifen (Nolvadex) prevents estrogen production that could stimulate the growth of tumor cells. Tamoxifen is an antiestrogen that may be used as an adjunct to surgery in postmenopausal women whose breast cancers are estrogen-receptor positive. It is also used as a palliative treatment for disseminated hormone-responsive breast cancer.**

1 and 3. Tamoxifen is not known to destroy cancer cells.
4. Tamoxifen does not cause calcium to deposit in bones.

Pregnancy Category: D
Client Need: Psychosocial Integrity

7 - 1 3

1. You will teach the client that the onset of insulin lispro injections (Humalog) is from 0.3 h to 0.5 h, the peak time is from 0.5 h to 2.5 h, and the duration time is from 3.0 h to 4.3 h. Humalog is a rapid-acting insulin whose onset, peak, and duration are faster than Regular insulin.

2. Humulin H is an intermediate-acting insulin with an onset between 1 and 2 h.

3. Iletin II insulin is an intermediate-acting insulin with an onset between 2 and 4 h.

4. Humulin U is a long-acting insulin with an onset between 4 and 6 h.

Pregnancy Category: NR

Client Need: Physiological Integrity

7 - 1 4

2. The client should receive 20 units of NPH and 12 units of Regular. Six units of Regular insulin should be added to the standard a.m. dosage of 6 units to manage the blood sugar pattern.

1. This dosage does not include the sliding scale coverage and would be an insufficient dosage at this time.

3. This is an overdosage of NPH and an insufficient dosage of Regular.

4. The Regular insulin dosage is correct, but the NPH dosage is an overdosage.

Pregnancy Category: NR

Client Need: Physiological Integrity

7 - 1 5

4. Glucocorticoid therapy may elevate serum glucose levels due to changes in carbohydrate metabolism. Gluconeogenesis (the formation of glucagon from noncarbohydrate sources) is affected by glucocorticoid therapy.

1. 210 mg/dl is an elevated, not low, serum glucose level.

2. Glucocorticoids do not stimulate the release of glucagon.

3. There is no indication that this client's pancreas is damaged.

Pregnancy Category: NR

Client Need: Physiological Integrity

7 - 1 6

③ **A client receiving NPH insulin at 7:00 a.m. is most likely to experience hypoglycemia (low blood glucose) during the insulin's peak time (between the noon and evening meals). A snack is usually given around 4:00 p.m. to prevent hypoglycemia. NPH insulin is an intermediate-acting insulin. Its onset is 1 to 4 hours, peak 6 to 12 hours, and duration 18 to 24 hours.**

1, 2, and 4. The peak effect of NPH insulin is 6 to 12 hours.

Pregnancy Category: NR

Client Need: Physiological Integrity

7 - 1 7

④ **Vasopressin (Pitressin) is an antidiuretic hormone replacement and may be given intramuscularly, subcutaneously, and nasally. Diabetes insipidus is a disorder of the pituitary gland. Normally, the pituitary produces the antidiuretic hormone that helps to concentrate urine. However, the pituitary gland of clients with diabetes insipidus does not produce the antidiuretic hormone, and clients may have a urinary output of 2 to 10 liters per day.**

1 and 2. Glipizide is a therapy for diabetes mellitus, not diabetes insipidus.

3. Vasopressin is not given intravenously.

Pregnancy Category: C

Client Need: Physiological Integrity

7 - 1 8

③ **It would be prudent to withhold the dosage of levothyroxine (Synthroid) in this instance and notify the physician. Clients on thyroid replacement such as levothyroxine (Synthroid) are at risk for pharmaceutically induced hyperthyroidism, whose symptoms include tachyarrhythmias.**

1. An adverse reaction to levothyroxine (Synthroid) is tachycardia. The nurse should withhold the medication, observe for other symptoms of toxicity, and notify the physician.

2. Cardiopulmonary resuscitation is not performed unless a client is not breathing and/or the heart is not beating.

4. Since levothyroxine (Synthroid) may cause tachycardia, it is unwise to anticipate an increase in the dosage.

Pregnancy Category: A

Client Need: Physiological Integrity

7 - 1 9

① **Prednisone should be tapered off gradually. Abrupt discontinuation of prednisone could lead to adrenal insufficiency. Because the adrenal glands are in part responsible for the release of steroids, steroid replacement suppresses adrenal activity. Abrupt withdrawal of exogenous steroids such as prednisone does not allow the body to adequately compensate for its new demands.**

2. Rapid withdrawal of prednisone could lead to adrenal insufficiency and should be avoided.

3. Prednisone causes gastrointestinal irritation and gastric ulcers and should be taken with food.

4. Prednisone causes sodium retention. These clients should receive a potassium supplement and a diet high in protein and calcium and low in sodium.

Pregnancy Category: C
Client Need: Health Promotion/Maintenance

7 - 2 0

① **Calcitonin-salmon (Calcimar) estrogen replacement and weight-bearing exercises increase calcium laydown in bones. Calcium supplements along with estrogen replacement and walking exercises improve bone stability by increasing available calcium for deposit in the bones and encouraging calcium laydown in response to bearing weight. Estrogen opposes bone resorption (release of calcium from the bones) and is presumed to be effective in treating estrogen deficiency-induced osteoporosis.**

2. The reduction of vasomotor instability ("hot flashes") is not related to preventing osteoporosis.

3. Osteoporosis is fairly inevitable with age, but a strong calcium matrix in the bone prolongs the time that the client can be free of osteoporotic fractures.

4. Estrogen enhances the coagulability of blood and is likely to increase the risk of clot formation.

Pregnancy Category: C
Client Need: Health Promotion/Maintenance

7 - 2 1

④ **If a client is able, carbohydrates by mouth should be encouraged following glucagon administration to avoid the likelihood of hypoglycemic rebound. Glucagon is a pancreatic hormone administered to manage severe hypoglycemia in situations in which administration of glucose is not possible. The hyperglycemic effect of this medication is only about 2 hours. Therefore, rebound hypoglycemia may occur.**

1. Glucagon is given to combat insulin shock (a condition caused by insulin overdose); therefore, you would not give insulin.

2. Carbohydrates by mouth are to be encouraged in alert clients to prevent hypoglycemic rebound.

3. There is no indication that the client needs an antacid such as sodium bicarbonate.

Pregnancy Category: B
Client Need: Health Promotion/Maintenance

7 - 2 2

② **Glucagon can increase the heart rate. Glucagon has a positive chronotropic effect (influencing the rate of heartbeat) and positive inotropic effect (influencing the force of muscular contractibility), which is most likely due to its impact on metabolic processes.**

1. Glucagon tends to increase the heart rate, not decrease it.
3. Glucagon is not administered to manage a hypertensive crisis.
4. Glucagon is a hormone used to treat hypoglycemia. It is not an antiviral agent.

Pregnancy Category: B

Client Need: Physiological Integrity

7 - 2 3

④ **The onset of long-acting insulins such as Ultralente is 4 to 6 hours, the peak action is 18 to 24 hours, and the duration is 36 hours.**

1. NPH insulin is intermediate-acting, not long-acting. The onset is 1 to 4 hours, the peak action is 6 to 12 hours, and the duration is 18 to 24 hours.
2. Long-acting insulin is available.
3. Long-acting insulin lasts up to 36 hours.

Pregnancy Category: NR

Client Need: Health Promotion/Maintenance

7 - 2 4

③ **You will explain to the client that insulin administered subcutaneously is the antidiabetic agent of choice for those who are NPO.**

1 and 4. The elevated glucose is probably due to infection and stress.
2. Oral medication cannot be given because the client is not to receive anything by mouth.

Pregnancy Category: NR

Client Need: Psychosocial Integrity

7 - 2 5

② **The prednisolone sodium (Predsol) retention enema should be withheld and the physician notified. Cushing's syndrome is an endocrine disorder associated with excessive steroids. This enema has systemic corticosteroid effects that may markedly worsen the symptoms of Cushing's syndrome.**

1. Prednisolone (Predsol) is contraindicated in Cushing's syndrome. However, when the enema is indicated, it is usually retained overnight.
3. Prednisolone enemas do have a systemic effect.
4. Bisacodyl enemas are not interchangeable with prednisolone enemas. Bisacodyl enemas manage constipation by stimulating peristalsis and would be contraindicated.

Pregnancy Category: C

Client Need: Health Promotion/Maintenance

7 - 2 6

① Chlorpropamide should not be used to treat Type 2 diabetes in alcoholic clients. Chlorpropamide is an oral medication used to treat Type 2 diabetes. It is a sulfonylurea and causes severe nausea and vomiting if the client drinks alcohol. Clients should also be taught to avoid cough syrups containing alcohol.

2, 3, and 4. Tolazamide, repaglinide, and glimepiride are all oral medications (sulfonylureas) used to treat Type 2 diabetes. Alcohol consumption is not prohibited with these sulfonylureas.

Pregnancy Category: C
Client Need: Physiological Integrity

7 - 2 7

① You will teach your client that lispro insulin (Humalog) has an onset of less than 30 minutes. Humalog is the fastest-acting insulin and is preferred when a rapid response is needed. This insulin lets the client "dose and eat."

2. Lispro (Humalog) peaks between 30 to 60 minutes. Regular insulin takes as long as 2 to 4 hours to peak.

3. Lispro (Humalog) lasts less than 6 hours. For this reason, it may be administered with an intermediate or long-acting insulin.

4. Lispro (Humalog) should be taken 10 to 15 minutes before eating. Clients should be taught that after taking Humalog, they need to eat within 15 minutes to avoid hypoglycemia.

Pregnancy Category: NR
Client Need: Physiological Integrity

7 - 2 8

③ The levothyroxine should be discontinued 4 weeks before the I 131 Uptake study is performed. The I 131 Uptake study requires the use of radioactive iodine. To eliminate incorrect results, all interfering factors, such as the administration of levothyroxine, should be withdrawn prior to the study.

1 and 2. If the I 131 Uptake study is scheduled only 2 to 3 weeks after the levothyroxine has been withdrawn, the results of the study will be invalid.

4. Levothyroxine should be withdrawn before the I 131 Uptake study. It is not necessary to wait longer than 4 weeks.

Pregnancy Category: A
Client Need: Health Promotion/Maintenance

Practice Test 8

Immunomodulation Agents

OVERVIEW

Immunomodulation (immunoregulation) refers to the effects of different chemical mediators, hormones, medications, or the immune system on foreign antigens. Immunomodulating agents (working through the body's immune system) will prevent, neutralize, or eliminate the effects of these foreign antigens.

Immunomodulating agents include:

- Antitoxins and antivenins
- Biological response modifiers
- Immune serums
- Immunosuppressants
- Vaccines and toxoids

ANTITOXINS AND ANTIVENINS

ANTITOXINS neutralize poisons, especially those generated by bacteria. Antitoxins produce antibodies in response to specific biologic toxins. Antitoxins are administered prophylactically and for therapeutic purposes.

Conditions treated with antitoxins include:

- Diphtheria
- Gas-gangrene
- Tetanus

ANTIVENINS are serums that contain antitoxins specific for animal or insect venoms. Antivenins are created from immunized animal serums and are administered to treat clients who have been poisoned by animal or insect venom.

Conditions treated with antivenins include:

- Poisonous spider bites
- Snakebites

BIOLOGICAL RESPONSE MODIFIERS

Biological response modifiers are a group of therapeutic interventions that modify the host response to various conditions or diseases. Biological response modifiers include cytokine, monoclonal antibodies, and vaccines that alter the interaction between clients and their tumors. Biological response modifiers promote antitumor mechanisms found naturally in the immune system.

Conditions treated with biological response modifiers include:

- Chronic hepatitis B
- Metastatic renal cell carcinoma
- Multiple sclerosis (to reduce exacerbations)

IMMUNE SERUMS

Serum from an animal that has been rendered immune to a pathogenic organism can be used to treat a person who has the disease caused by that pathogenic organism. Immune serums contain antibodies for specific antigens.

Conditions treated with immune serums include:

- Tetanus, in clients who have not been immunized with tetanus toxoid but have been exposed to the tetanus pathogen
- Pertussis (whooping cough), as both prophylaxis and treatment

IMMUNOSUPPRESSANTS

Immunosuppressants prevent the formation of immune responses—that is, they suppress the body's natural immune response to antigens.

Conditions treated with immunosuppressants include:

- Organ rejection (heart, kidney, liver, pancreas) as prophylaxis

VACCINES AND TOXOIDS

A VACCINE is a suspension of an infectious agent or some part of an infectious agent administered to create a resistance to that infection. Vaccines are grouped into classes:

(1) Vaccines containing live attenuated (weakened) infectious organisms, such as the vaccine to prevent poliomyelitis.

(2) Vaccines containing infectious agents that can be destroyed by physical or chemical means.

(3) Vaccines containing soluble toxins of microorganisms (i.e., toxoids) used in the prevention of diphtheria and tetanus.

(4) Vaccines containing substances extracted from infectious agents (i.e., the capsular polysaccharides extracted from pneumococci).

Conditions treated with vaccines include:

- Mumps
- Poliomyelitis
- Rabies
- Rubella
- Smallpox

TOXOIDS are toxins that have been treated to destroy their toxicity but remain capable of inducing the formation of antibodies by injection. They are sometimes called anatoxins.

Conditions treated with toxoids include:

- Diphtheria
- Tetanus

Practice Test 8

Questions

8 - 1

A client with acquired immunodeficiency syndrome (AIDS) has Kaposi's sarcoma. Interferon alfa-2b (Intron A) 30 million units 3 times a week has been prescribed. After initial treatment, the client states that a friend has leftover interferon (Roferon) and asks if it can be substituted. The nurse will inform the client that:

1. the medicines are interchangeable.
2. different brands of interferon may not be equivalent and may require different dosages.
3. one brand cannot be substituted with another due to differences in chemical components.
4. it is not wise to use old drugs, since their potency may be questionable.

8 - 2

Which of the following information would preclude a prospective donor from giving blood?

1. hemoglobin 14.0 gm/dL
2. body weight of 72 kg
3. blood pressure of 150/90 mmHg
4. received rubella vaccine in the previous 2 weeks

8 - 3

A gravida I, 30-week gestation, is Rh-negative and her husband is Rh-positive. As you speak to her about RhoGam, she expresses concern for the baby she is now carrying. Your reply is based on your knowledge that:

1. RhoGam will destroy any antibodies formed.
2. this baby will be Rh-negative.
3. this baby can be treated with blood transfusions at birth.
4. antibodies are not formed until exposure to the antigen.

8 - 4

Following your client's liver transplant, a prescription was written for cyclosporine (Sandimmune) 600 mg oral solution to be given daily. Prior to discharge, the client will be taught to:

1. take the medication from a plastic medicine cup.
2. take a double dose if previous dosage was omitted.
3. report any changes in kidney function.
4. receive flu vaccinations in case of outbreaks.

8 - 5

The mother of an 8-month-old infant telephones the clinic and states that her child is scheduled to receive immunizations today but is sick and has a fever. The nurse should instruct the mother to:

1. bring the child to the clinic anyway because immunizations should be kept on schedule.
2. skip this set of immunizations and resume the schedule with the 15-month immunizations.
3. bring the child to the clinic to receive the immunizations as soon as the child is well.
4. bring the child to the clinic anyway because the immunizations will help the child to recover from the present illness more quickly.

8 - 6

A client receiving the initial dosage of the LYMErix vaccine asks you, "How many more dosages do I have to take?" You will tell the client that the entire dosing schedule consists of:

1. 3 intramuscular dosages given over the course of 1 year.
2. 2 intramuscular dosages given over the course of 6 months.
3. 3 oral dosages given at 4-month intervals.
4. 2 subcutaneous dosages given at 3-month intervals.

8 - 7

Which one of the following immunizations may be administered to a pregnant woman?

1. rubeola
2. mumps
3. rubella
4. recombinant hepatitis B vaccine

8 - 8

A client comes to the outpatient clinic and tells the nurse, "I have never had a flu shot, but I would like to have one this year." What information elicited from the client would indicate that the influenza virus vaccine should not be given?

1. The client has chronic obstructive pulmonary disease.
2. The client has been exposed to the measles.
3. The client has a hypersensitivity to egg whites.
4. The client is anemic.

8 - 9

How often should people who have had their initial tetanus immunizations receive a booster?

1. every year
2. every 2 years
3. every 5 years
4. every 10 years

8 - 1 0

An immunocompromised client tells you, "I have been exposed to the shingles. Is there anything I can do to avoid infection?" Your best response would be:

1. "There are antiviral medications that can be administered."
2. "The varicella-zoster immunoglobulin can prevent infection."
3. "You cannot be protected from infection once you have been exposed."
4. "Should you become infected, there are analgesics to relieve the pain."

Practice Test 8

Answers, Rationales, and Explanations

8 - 1

② **The nurse will inform the client that different brands of interferon (a biological response modifier) may not be equivalent and may require different dosages.**

1. Different brands of interferon cannot be interchanged due to equivalency and dosage differences.
3. The difference is in the equivalency and dosages, not in the chemical composition.
4. There is no indication that the drug is old or has questionable potency.

Pregnancy Category: C
Client Need: Physiological Integrity

8 - 2

④ **Blood should not be donated by a person who has had a rubella vaccine within the previous 2 weeks. The live organisms used in the rubella vaccine (Meruvax II) may be passed from donor to recipient through a blood transfusion. A waiting period of 2 months is recommended before a person vaccinated with the rubella vaccine should donate blood.**

1. A hemoglobin of 14.0 gm/dl is within the normal range and would not preclude a donor from giving blood.
2. A body weight of 72 kg (158 pounds) would not preclude donating blood.
3. A blood pressure of 150/90 mmHg would not preclude donating blood.

Pregnancy Category: Rubella vaccine, C
Client Need: Health Promotion/Maintenance

8 - 3

④ **Antibodies are not formed until exposure to antigens. RhoGam (an immune serum) promotes lysis of fetal Rh-positive blood cells that have entered the maternal circulation. As a consequence, antibodies to Rh-positive blood cells are not formed. Major exposure to the fetus's Rh-positive blood occurs after separation of the placenta. Therefore, RhoGam should be given to the mother within 72 hours after delivery.**

1. RhoGam promotes lysis of fetal Rh-positive blood cells that are exposed to maternal circulation. It does not destroy antibodies.
2. To be incompatible, the baby's blood will have to be Rh-positive.
3. The first baby is not usually affected, since major exposure to fetal Rh-positive blood occurs with separation of the placenta.

Pregnancy Category: C
Client Need: Health Promotion/Maintenance

8 - 4

③ **Clients receiving cyclosporine (Sandimmune) should be taught to report changes in kidney function. Cyclosporine is an immunosuppressant prescribed for the treatment and prevention of cardiac, hepatic, and renal transplant rejection. Cyclosporine is nephrotoxic (damages kidney cells) and signs of nephrotoxicity should be reported. Blood urea nitrogen and creatinine should be monitored, especially during the first few months of therapy, to detect impaired renal function.**

1. Glass containers should be used because cyclosporine has a tendency to adhere to plastic, altering the dosage.

2. Dosage should not be doubled since this may cause overdosage. Teach the client to take the medication at the same time every day to avoid forgetting.

4. Clients may have a decreased immune response because cyclosporine is an immunosuppressant. Therefore, vaccinations should be postponed.

Pregnancy Category: C

Client Need: Health Promotion/Maintenance

8 - 5

③ **Children with a fever should not receive immunizations. Immunizations should be given as soon as possible after the illness is past. Contraindications for receiving immunizations include febrile illnesses, seizure disorder (pertussis component), immunosuppression, malignancy, prior reaction to an immunization, and recent gamma globulin. Conditions that do not contraindicate immunization include chronic illness and non-febrile acute illness.**

1. Immunizing children who are sick and have a fever could compromise their immune systems further.

2. Immunization should not be skipped because giving immunizations in a series and at predetermined intervals provides protection gradually without compromising the child's health.

4. Immunizations protect children from specific diseases. To give children immunizations when they are sick could compromise their immune systems further.

Pregnancy Category: NR

Client Need: Health Promotion/Maintenance

8 - 6

① **You will explain to clients receiving the LYMErix vaccine that the dosing schedule consists of 3 intramuscular injections given over the course of 1 year. After the initial injection, another injection is given in 1 month, followed by the third (last) injection 11 months later.**

2. Three intramuscular injections are given over the course of 1 year.

3 and 4. The dosages are given intramuscularly, not orally, and they are given over the course of 1 year, not 6 months.

Pregnancy Category: C

Client Need: Health Promotion/Maintenance

8 - 7

---

④ **The recombinant hepatitis B vaccine may be given to a pregnant woman. Vaccines containing killed viruses may be administered during pregnancy. Vaccines containing killed viruses include those for tetanus, diphtheria, recombinant hepatitis B, and rabies.**

1, 2, and 3. Immunizations containing live or attenuated live viruses, such as those for rubeola, rubella, and mumps, are contraindicated during pregnancy because they can be teratogenic; that is, they may cause the development of abnormal embryonic structures that result in severe fetal deformities.

Pregnancy Category: Immunizations containing live viruses are contraindicated.

Client Need: Health Promotion/Maintenance

8 - 8

---

③ **Clients who have a hypersensitivity to egg whites should not be injected with the influenza virus vaccine because preparation of the vaccine involves exposure to egg whites.**

1. The annual influenza virus vaccine is recommended for clients with chronic disorders of the pulmonary and cardiovascular systems. These people are more likely to contract the flu and also more likely to become incapacitated by it.

2. Having been exposed to the measles would not interfere with a client receiving an influenza virus vaccine.

4. Clients who are anemic should receive the influenza virus vaccine. They are in a high-risk group for contracting the flu.

Pregnancy Category: C

Client Need: Health Promotion/Maintenance

8 - 9

---

④ **After the initial tetanus immunization, clients should receive a booster every 10 years.**

1. It is not necessary to have a booster of tetanus toxoid every year. The initial immunization should protect a person for 10 years.

2. The initial tetanus immunization will protect a person for 10 years.

3. A booster of tetanus toxoid is necessary if it has been 5 years since the last immunization and the client has a major contaminated wound. Otherwise, the initial immunization will protect a person for 10 years.

Pregnancy Category: C

Client Need: Health Promotion/Maintenance

8 - 1 0

② **People who have been exposed to shingles can receive the varicella-zoster immuno-globulin within 72 hours of exposure and be protected from the infection.**

1. Antiviral medications such as Famvir are given to treat clients who have shingles. Antivirals will not prevent the shingles.

3. Protection is available (varicella-zoster immunoglobulin-VZIG) that can prevent those who have been exposed to shingles from becoming infected.

4. Analgesics are available to treat the pain associated with shingles; however, analgesics will not prevent shingles.

Pregnancy Category: C

Client Need: Health Promotion/Maintenance

Practice Test 9

Autonomic Nervous System Agents

OVERVIEW

The autonomic nervous system is composed of the sympathetic and parasympathetic nervous systems. Autonomic nervous system agents are administered to treat, prevent, and inhibit conditions associated with these two systems.

Autonomic nervous system agents include:

- Adrenergics (sympathomimetics)
- Adrenergic blockers (sympatholytics)
- Anticholinergics (parasympatholytics)
- Cholinergics (parasympathomimetics)
- Neuromuscular blockers
- Skeletal muscle relaxants

ADRENERGICS (SYMPATHOMIMETICS)

Adrenergics (sympathomimetics) are nerve fibers that when stimulated release epinephrine at their endings. Adrenergics generally produce one or more of the following reactions:

- Wakefulness, rapid reaction to stimuli, quickened reflexes
- Constriction of blood vessels, decrease in gastric motility
- Increase in heart rate
- Increased use of glucose along with release of fatty acids from the adipose tissues

Conditions treated with adrenergics include:

- Cardiac decompensation (adrenergics increase cardiac output)
- Shock (adrenergics restore blood pressure in acute hypotensive states)
- Adrenergics are also administered to increase blood perfusion to vital organs (e.g., kidneys)

ADRENERGIC BLOCKERS (SYMPATHOLYTICS)

Adrenergic blockers oppose or inhibit adrenergic nerve function. They can cause antagonistic effects of serotonin $5HT_2$ receptors and inhibit reuptake of norepinephrine.

Conditions treated with adrenergic blockers include:

- Vascular headaches, to prevent or abort
- Migraine headaches, to prevent or abort

ANTICHOLINERGICS (PARASYMPATHOLYTICS)

Anticholinergics (parasympatholytics) mimic the action of the sympathetic nervous system. The sympathetic nervous system coordinates actions that are used to cope with stress. Some effects of sympathetic stimulation include thick, odoriferous secretions, increased heart rate, dilated bronchi, and increased mental activity.

Conditions treated with anticholinergics (parasympatholytics) include:

- Peptic ulcers, as adjunct therapy
- Allergic rhinitis
- Renal colic
- Spastic states

CHOLINERGICS (PARASYMPATHOMIMETICS)

Cholinergics mimic the activity of the parasympathetic nervous system. The parasympathetic nerves are involuntary autonomic nerves that help regulate body functions. The parasympathetic nervous system is associated with conservation and restoration of energy stores. Some effects of parasympathetic stimulation include: Constriction of pupils, contraction of smooth muscle in the alimentary canal, constriction of bronchioles, slowing of the heart rate, and increased secretion by all the glands (except the sweat glands).

Conditions treated with cholinergics (parasympathomimetics) include:

- Acute painful musculoskeletal conditions
- Cholinergics are also administered as an antidote for nondepolarizing neuromuscular blockers.
- Acute postoperative/postpartum nonobstructive (functional) urine retention
- Myasthenia gravis

NEUROMUSCULAR BLOCKERS

Neuromuscular blockers provide skeletal muscle relaxation by antagonizing (interrupting) the effects of acetylcholine, which in turn blocks neuromuscular transmission.

Neuromuscular blockers include:

- Mivacurium chloride (Mivacron)
- Pancuronium bromide (Pavulon)
- Succinylcholine chloride (Anectine)

Neuromuscular blockers are administered to:

- Facilitate endotracheal intubation
- Facilitate mechanical ventilation
- Provide muscle relaxation during surgery

SKELETAL MUSCLE RELAXANTS

Skeletal muscle relaxants are administered to relieve acute muscle pain. Although the action of skeletal muscle relaxants is not fully understood, they are thought to relieve pain by their sedative effects and their ability to reduce transmission of nerve impulses from the spinal cord to the skeletal muscles.

Skeletal muscle relaxants include:

- Diazepam (Valium)
- Cyclobenzaprine (Flexeril)
- Methocarbamol (Robaxin)

Conditions treated with skeletal muscle relaxants include:

- Muscle spasms
- Acute painful musculoskeletal conditions

Practice Test 9

Questions

9 - 1

A client has developed acute renal insufficiency following antibiotic therapy. A dopamine (Intropin) infusion is administered to restore renal function. The mechanism of dopamine's therapeutic action includes:

1. increasing renal perfusion.
2. lowering blood pressure.
3. increasing cardiac output.
4. increasing renal excretion of water and electrolytes.

9 - 2

Your client is experiencing excessive salivation following a partial glossectomy. You will anticipate a prescription for:

1. acetylcholine.
2. atropine.
3. pilocarpine.
4. bethanechol.

9 - 3

The nurse observes that a client with low back pain has increased mobility and has begun to participate in activities of daily living. Which of the following medications would most likely be responsible for these behaviors?

1. diazepam (Valium)
2. dronabinol (Marinol)
3. clonazepam (Klonopin)
4. carbamazepine (Tegretol)

9 - 4

Which of the following medications may be given to a client experiencing severe lower back muscle pain?

1. torsemide (Demadex)
2. fludarabine phosphate (Fludara)
3. cyclobenzaprine (Flexeril)
4. diltiazem (Cardizem)

9 - 5

Methocarbamol (Robaxin) 1 gram intravenous has been prescribed for your client's muscle spasms. When administering this medication, you will:

1. infuse the drug rapidly since Robaxin's stability is short-lived.
2. inject the drug slowly after placing the client in a supine position.
3. have the client participate in exercise following drug administration.
4. instruct the client that light-headedness and drowsiness are expected after administration of this drug.

9 - 6

You are to administer bethanechol chloride (Urecholine) to a client experiencing acute postoperative nonobstructive urine retention. Prior to administering this drug, you will:

1. gather and prepare the necessary IV equipment.
2. have acetylcholine injectable available and ready to administer.
3. administer an SQ test dose of the medication.
4. teach the client that the drug's effects are usually felt within 3 to 4 hours of administration.

9 - 7

Your client is receiving pseudoephedrine sulfate (Afrin) 120 mg extended-release capsules daily to treat nasal congestion. You will teach the client:

1. not to crush or break the extended-release capsules.
2. to take the medication as close to bedtime as possible.
3. to anticipate a sedative effect.
4. that the medication may be taken concurrently with antihypertensives.

9 - 8

Your client is scheduled for an appendectomy. You will administer atropine sulfate 0.4 mg IM preoperatively. You know the purpose of this medication is to block cardiac vagal reflexes and:

1. facilitate symptomatic relief of bradycardia.
2. treat functional gastrointestinal disorders, such as appendicitis.
3. diminish secretions.
4. decrease the number of gastrointestinal bacteria.

9 - 9

Following an automobile accident, your client experienced muscle spasms and was placed on cyclobenzaprine hydrochloride (Flexeril) 10 mg tid over a 3-week period. You will teach the client to:

1. notify the physician should the side effect of diarrhea occur.
2. continue all activities as usual.
3. consume alcohol and OTC cold and allergy remedies in moderation.
4. report any urinary hesitation or retention.

9 - 1 0

Your client experienced a positive reaction to a Tensilon test. Thereafter, the client was placed on the drug pyridostigmine bromide (Mestinon). You know this drug has been prescribed to treat:

1. multiple sclerosis.
2. Alzheimer's disease.
3. Parkinson's disease.
4. myasthenia gravis.

Practice Test 9

Answers, Rationales, and Explanations

9 - 1

①   **Dopamine (Intropin) causes renal vasodilation, thus increasing renal perfusion. Dopamine is an adrenergic (sympathomimetic) that stimulates receptors of the sympathic nervous system, facilitating vasodilation and thereby improving perfusion to vital organs.**

2.   With improved renal function, the client's blood pressure will return to normal (decrease) as an indirect action of dopamine (Intropin).

3.   Dopamine (Intropin) does not directly improve cardiac output.

4.   With improved renal function, water and electrolyte excretion will increase; however, this is not the primary action of dopamine (Intropin) in this situation.

Pregnancy Category: C

Client Need: Physiological Integrity

9 - 2

②   **A prescription for atropine will be anticipated. Atropine is an anticholinergic (blocks impulses through the parasympathetic nerves) that produces an antisecretory action (vagolytic effect), decreasing perspiration, lacrimation (tears), and secretions from the nose, mouth, pharynx, and bronchi.**

1, 3, and 4.   Acetylcholine, pilocarpine, and bethanechol are all cholinergic drugs (parasympathomimetics) and are associated with an increase in respiratory tract fluids. Administering these drugs would potentiate the drooling (salivation).

Pregnancy Category: C

Client Need: Physiological Integrity

9 - 3

①   **Diazepam (Valium) and methocarbamol (Robaxin) are often prescribed for management of pain associated with muscle spasms. As pain relief is achieved, clients increase their activity. Diazepam (Valium) is a central nervous system anti-anxiety agent effective in treating muscle spasms. It is also given as a preoperative sedation and as an adjunct in the treatment of seizure disorders.**

2.   Marinol (Dronabinol) is an antiemetic (cannabinoid) and is the main psychoactive ingredient of marijuana. It is used to treat nausea and vomiting associated with chemotherapy. It does not directly affect muscle spasms.

3 and 4.   Clonazepam (Klonopin) and carbamazepine (Tegretol) are anticonvulsant drugs and do not directly affect muscle spasms.

Pregnancy Category: D

Client Need: Health Promotion/Maintenance

9 - 4

③ **Cyclobenzaprine (Flexeril) is an autonomic nervous system skeletal muscle relaxant. Its action is not clearly understood, but it relieves muscle spasms.**

1. Torsemide (Demadex) is a loop diuretic and does not affect muscle pain.
2. Fludarabine phosphate (Fludara) is an antimetabolite and does not affect muscle pain.
4. Diltiazem (Cardizem) is an antianginal/antiarrhythmic and does not affect skeletal muscle pain.

Pregnancy Category: B

Client Need: Health Promotion/Maintenance

9 - 5

② **To minimize orthostatic hypotension and other adverse side effects, an intravenous injection of methocarbamol (Robaxin) should be administered slowly with the client in a supine position.**

1. Robaxin administered intravenously should be infused slowly since rapid administration is known to cause bradycardia, hypotension, and dizziness.
3. It is not advisable to encourage activity following the intravenous administration of Robaxin since this medication may cause bradycardia, hypotension, and dizziness.
4. Light-headedness and drowsiness could be due to hypotension, an adverse side effect of Robaxin. They are not expected outcomes.

Pregnancy Category: NR

Client Need: Safe, Effective Care Environment

9 - 6

③ **A test dose of bethanechol chloride (Urecholine) will always be given SQ to determine the minimal effective dose. A 2.5-mg SQ dose is given and then repeated every 15 to 30 minutes for a total of 4 doses.**

1. Bethanechol chloride should never be given IV or IM since it could cause circulatory collapse.
2. Injectable atropine (an anticholinergic) should be available to provide circulatory support if needed—not acetylcholine.
4. The effects of bethanechol chloride (Urecholine) are felt within 30 to 90 minutes.

Pregnancy Category: C

Client Need: Health Promotion/Maintenance

9 - 7

(1) **You will teach the client that extended-release capsules should not be crushed or broken. Extended-release capsules are designed to release their medication gradually. After the capsule dissolves, the granules dissolve at different rates. This reduces the number of dosages administered per day.**

2. Sympathomimetics, such as Afrin, should not be taken within 2 hours of bedtime because they may cause insomnia.

3. Sympathomimetics may cause a client to experience unusual restlessness, not sedation.

4. Pseudoephedrine sulfate (Afrin) should not be taken concurrently with antihypertensives because it could cause a hypertensive crisis.

Pregnancy Category: C
Client Need: Physiological Integrity

9 - 8

(3) **In addition to blocking cardiac vagal reflexes, atropine sulfate is given preoperatively to diminish secretions that could otherwise be aspirated and precipitate the development of postoperative pneumonia.**

1. Atropine sulfate may be given to treat symptomatic bradycardia. However, it is not given preoperatively for this purpose.

2. Atropine sulfate is given to treat peptic ulcer disease as well as other functional gastrointestinal disorders such as irritable bowel syndrome. However, it is not given preoperatively to treat these conditions.

4. An anti-infective would be given to decrease gastrointestinal bacteria, not an anticholinergic.

Pregnancy Category: C
Client Need: Health Promotion/Maintenance

9 - 9

(4) **You will teach the client to report any urinary hesitation or retention. Cyclobenzaprine hydrochloride (Flexeril) is a skeletal muscle relaxant and should be used cautiously in clients who have a history of urinary retention, acute angle-closure glaucoma, and increased intraocular pressure.**

1. Constipation, not diarrhea, is a gastrointestinal tract reaction to cyclobenzaprine hydrochloride (Flexeril). Constipation is usually treated by increasing fluid intake and administering a stool softener.

2. Clients receiving cyclobenzaprine should be taught to avoid activities that require alertness until their reaction to the drug's CNS effects are known.

3. Alcohol, over-the-counter (OTC) cold and allergy remedies, and CNS depressants should not be combined with cyclobenzaprine hydrochloride (Flexeril) since they potentiate each other's effects.

Pregnancy Category: B
Client Need: Health Promotion/Maintenance

9 - 1 0

④ **You know that pyridostigmine bromide (Mestinon) is administered to treat the symptoms of myasthenia gravis (a condition affecting the voluntary muscles). Symptoms include: Muscle weakness and fatigability. To confirm a tentative diagnosis of myasthenia gravis, a Tensilon test is given. If the client responds positively to an intravenous injection of edrophonium (Tensilon), then it can be determined that the client has myasthenia gravis.**

1. Multiple sclerosis is not treated with Mestinon. Drugs associated with the treatment of multiple sclerosis include: Baclofen, dantrolene, glatiramer acetate, interferon, and prednisone.

2. Alzheimer's disease is not treated with Mestinon. It is treated with drugs such as donepezil (Aricept).

3. Parkinson's disease is not treated with Mestinon. It is treated with drugs such as levodopa.

Pregnancy Category: C
Client Need: Health Promotion/Maintenance

Practice Test 10

Central Nervous System Agents

OVERVIEW

Central nervous system agents affect the functioning of nervous tissue. Many of these agents penetrate the blood-brain barrier and exert their effects directly on the brain and spinal cord.

Central nervous system agents include:

- Antianxiety agents
- Anticonvulsives
- Antidepressants
- Antiparkinsonians
- Antipsychotics
- Central nervous system stimulants
- Narcotics and opioid analgesics
- Nonnarcotic analgesics and antipyretics
- Nonsteroidal anti-inflammatory substances
- Sedative hypnotics

ANTIANXIETY AGENTS

Antianxiety agents are used in the short-term treatment of anxiety. Long-term use of antianxiety agents is not recommended because of the potential for drug dependency associated with serious withdrawal symptoms. Some antianxiety drugs are controlled substances.

Antianxiety agents include:

- Alprazolam (Xanax)
- Diazepam (Valium)
- Midazolam hydrochloride (Versed)

Conditions treated with antianxiety agents include:

- Acute alcohol withdrawal
- Seizure disorders, as adjunct therapy
- Mild to moderate anxiety
- Panic attacks
- Antianxiety agents may also be administered before endoscopic procedures to reduce client anxiety.

ANTICONVULSIVES

Anticonvulsives manage convulsions and seizures. Most anticonvulsives are administered in the treatment of specific types of seizure, such as generalized tonic-clonic seizures, partial seizures, and status epilepticus.

Anticonvulsives include:

- Phenobarbital (Solfoton)
- Phenobarbital sodium (sodium luminal)
- Phenytoin (Dilantin)

Conditions treated with anticonvulsives include:

- Epilepsy
- Febrile seizures
- Generalized tonic-clonic seizures
- Seizures associated with preeclampsia or eclampsia

ANTIDEPRESSANTS

Antidepressants are psychotherapeutic substances used in the management of various types of depression as well as in depression associated with anxiety. Antidepressants fall into two major divisions:

(1) monoamine oxidase inhibitors (MAOIs) (2) tricyclic antidepressants

MONOAMINE OXIDASE INHIBITORS (MAOIs) include:

- Fluoxetine (Prozac)
- Phenelzine sulfate (Nardil)

TRICYCLIC ANTIDEPRESSANTS include:

- Amitriptyline (Elavil)
- Clomipramine hydrochloride (Anafranil)
- Doxepin (Sinequan)

Conditions treated with antidepressants include:

- Depression
- Obsessive-compulsive disorders

ANTIPARKINSONIANS

Antiparkinsonians treat the symptoms of parkinsonism (paralysis agitans); i.e., tremors, muscle rigidity and weakness, masklike face, difficulty chewing and swallowing, and a shuffling gait. Antiparkinsonians also treat many of the symptoms of extrapyramidal disorders.

Antiparkinsonians include:

- Carbidopa (Lodosyn)
- Levodopa (Larodopa)

Conditions treated with antiparkinsonians include:

- Drug-induced extrapyramidal disorders; i.e., tremors, chorea, athetosis (irregular twisting of hands), and dystonia
- Parkinsonism

ANTIPSYCHOTICS

Antipsychotics are used in the management of various psychotic conditions. A few antipsychotics have specific uses; for example, lithium carbonate is used to treat manic-depressive psychosis.

Antipsychotics include:

- Haloperidol (Haldol)
- Thioridazine (Mellaril)

Conditions treated with antipsychotics include:

- Behavioral problems associated with chronic organic mental syndrome
- Nonpsychotic behavioral disorders
- Psychotic disorders; i.e., schizophrenia
- Motor and phonic tics in clients with Tourette syndrome

CENTRAL NERVOUS SYSTEM STIMULANTS

Central nervous system (CNS) agents temporarily increase the functional activity of the brain and spinal cord along with the nerves and organs that control voluntary and involuntary acts.

CNS stimulants include:

- Amphetamines
- Anorexiants
- Analeptics

AMPHETAMINES stimulate the central nervous system. Prolonged use of amphetamines may cause drug dependency. Amphetamines are administered to treat conditions such as narcolepsy and obesity.

ANALEPTICS stimulate the central nervous system. They are administered most frequently to treat clients who have been poisoned or have depressed the central nervous system with drugs such as barbiturates.

ANOREXIANTS are substances that suppress the appetite by stimulating the central nervous system. These substances are administered primarily to treat obesity as a short-term adjunct.

CNS stimulants include:

- Amphetamine sulfate
- Doxapram hydrochloride (Dopram)
- Dextroamphetamine sulfate (Dexedrine)
- Methylphenidate (Ritalin)

Conditions treated with CNS stimulants include:

- Exogenous obesity (obesity due to overeating), as adjunct therapy
- Attention deficit disorder with hyperactivity
- Narcolepsy (uncontrolled bouts of sleep)
- CNS stimulants are also administered to stimulate the respiratory system postanesthesia.

NARCOTICS AND OPIOID ANALGESICS

Narcotics are capable of depressing the central nervous system. They relieve pain and produce sleep. Opioid analgesics are narcotics derived from opium (poppy plants). Narcotics and opioid analgesics are controlled substances.

Narcotics and opioid analgesics include:

- Codeine (Codeine sulfate)
- Morphine sulfate (Roxanol)
- Meperidine hydrochloride (Demerol)

Conditions treated with narcotics and opioids include:

- Moderate to severe pain

NONNARCOTIC ANALGESICS AND ANTIPYRETICS

Nonnarcotic analgesics relieve pain. Unlike narcotic analgesics, they do not cause physical dependency. There are two groups of nonnarcotic analgesics:

(1) salicylates (various forms of a white crystalline acid derived from phenol), including aspirin and substances related to aspirin

(2) nonsalicylates, including ibuprofen and indomethacin

Nonnarcotic analgesics and antipyretics include:

- Acetaminophen (Tylenol)
- Aspirin (ASA)

Conditions treated with nonnarcotic analgesics and antipyretics include:

- Elevated body temperature
- Rheumatoid arthritis
- Mild to moderate pain
- Rheumatic fever

NONSTEROIDAL ANTI-INFLAMMATORY SUBSTANCES

The nonsteroidal anti-inflammatory substances (NSAIDs) are prostaglandin inhibitors. They have, to varying degrees, analgesic, antipyretic, and anti-inflammatory effects. Nonsteroidal anti-inflammatory substances are most effectively used to relieve pain and inflammation.

Nonsteroidal anti-inflammatory substances include:

- Ibuprofen (Motrin)
- Tolmetin sodium (Tolectin)
- Indomethacin (Indocin)

Conditions treated with nonsteroidal anti-inflammatory substances include:

- Acute painful shoulder
- Rheumatoid and osteoarthritis
- Primary dysmenorrhea

SEDATIVE HYPNOTICS

Sedatives produce a soothing, tranquilizing effect. Some are controlled substances. Sedative hypnotics fall into three divisions: general, nervous, and vascular.

Sedative hypnotics include:

- Chloral hydrate (Noctec)
- Secobarbital sodium (Seconal)
- Pentobarbital (Nembutal)

Conditions treated with sedative hypnotics include:

- Insomnia
- Sedative hypnotics are also administered for preoperative sedation and sedation in general.

Practice Test 10

Questions

1 0 - 1

Which of the following medications might be used in the treatment of mood disorders?

1. digoxin (Lanoxin)
2. ranitidine (Zantac)
3. atenolol (Tenormin)
4. fluoxetine (Prozac)

1 0 - 2

Your postoperative client has received intrathecal morphine. Nursing actions for this client will include:

1. notifying the physician if the client's respiratory rate falls below 6.
2. instructing your client to avoid coughing and deep breathing for 24 hours.
3. keeping flumazenil (Romazicon) available.
4. monitoring the respiratory rate and pattern at least hourly for 24 hours.

1 0 - 3

A client with Parkinson's disease is experiencing increasing functional impairment and is to be given carbidopa-levodopa (Sinemet). The nurse explains that the therapeutic action of this drug is to:

1. replace dopamine normally present in the central nervous system.
2. suppress dopamine production in the central nervous system.
3. reduce spasticity of voluntary muscles.
4. slow nerve impulse transmission in the central nervous system.

1 0 - 4

A client is experiencing sickle-cell crisis. Which of the following medications do you anticipate administering?

1. antacids
2. antiarrhythmics
3. antihistamines
4. analgesics

1 0 - 5

A client with pneumonia is complaining of pain. The client is also febrile. Which of the following medications is both an analgesic and an antipyretic?

1. ibuprofen (Motrin)
2. meperidine (Demerol)
3. promethazine (Phenergan)
4. ampicillin (Omnipen)

1 0 - 6

Your client is experiencing cardiac chest pains. Morphine (Duramorph) has been prescribed. You know this is an appropriate treatment because:

1. morphine directly dissolves blood clots.
2. morphine is a hallucinogenic.
3. morphine stimulates the central nervous system.
4. morphine improves circulation and relieves pain.

1 0 - 7

A client with severe rheumatoid arthritis is to receive methotrexate (Rheumatrex) 10 mg by mouth weekly. Which other drugs used to treat this condition can increase methotrexate toxicity?

1. nonsteroidal anti-inflammatory agents
2. muscle relaxants
3. steroidal anti-inflammatory agents
4. iron supplements

1 0 - 8

A client with Parkinson's disease is experiencing impaired physical functioning and is receiving dopamine (levodopa). Which of the following instructions should your teaching plan include regarding the potential side effects of levodopa?

1. Rise slowly from a supine to a sitting position.
2. Take multivitamin supplements.
3. Avoid operating moving vehicles.
4. Follow a high-protein diet.

10-9

A 15-year-old is brought to the Emergency Department after ingesting 50 aceta-minophen (Tylenol) tablets. The nurse will expect the plan of care to include all but one of the following:

1. the administration of Mucomyst
2. monitoring for prolonged bleeding time
3. monitoring for hypoglycemia
4. monitoring for liver and renal function

10-10

A client experiencing tendinitis will receive the most relief with which of the following medications?

1. acetaminophen (Tylenol)
2. ibuprofen (Motrin)
3. liotrix (Euthroid)
4. theophylline (Theobid)

10-11

A client with sudden and acute onset of renal calculi would benefit from which category of medication?

1. analgesics
2. antiarrhythmics
3. diuretics
4. antivirals

10-12

To maximize the efficacy of levodopa (Dopar), you will instruct your client to take the medication:

1. with food and before major activities of the day.
2. before bedtime, to reduce daytime sedation.
3. only when symptoms are bothersome.
4. after meals, to reduce gastrointestinal irritation.

1 0 - 1 3

The physician prescribed fentanyl (Duragesic), a 25-mcg transdermal patch to be applied daily for a client experiencing chronic pain. The nurse will:

1. question the dosage of the drug.
2. expect full analgesia effects within 1 hour.
3. anticipate hypertensive and tachypneic side effects.
4. apply the patch to the same area consistently.

1 0 - 1 4

Which of the following medications would be used in the treatment of tonic-clonic seizure?

1. divalproex sodium (Depakote)
2. ranitidine (Zantac)
3. digoxin (Lanoxin)
4. captopril (Capoten)

1 0 - 1 5

Which of the following would be helpful in relieving the pain associated with a fracture?

1. furosemide (Lasix)
2. ranitidine (Zantac)
3. ketorolac (Toradol)
4. bretylium (Bretylol)

1 0 - 1 6

A client has been taking ethinyl estradiol (Estinyl) and is to begin taking phenytoin (Dilantin) for a seizure disorder. What change, if any, do you anticipate in this client's ethinyl estradiol dosage?

1. The dosage will be increased.
2. There will be no change in the dosage.
3. The dosage will be decreased.
4. The dosage will be discontinued immediately.

1 0 - 1 7

A client experiencing tendinitis is to receive naproxen sodium (Naprelan) 500 mg, po, bid. You will teach the client that this medication:

1. is a sedating narcotic.
2. should be taken with food.
3. is the drug of choice for people with peptic ulcer disease who require analgesia.
4. must be taken on an empty stomach to be effective.

1 0 - 1 8

An alcoholic is experiencing delirium tremens (DTs). You would anticipate a prescription for:

1. Stelazine.
2. Antabuse.
3. Librium.
4. Prolixin.

1 0 - 1 9

Your client is receiving trihexyphenidyl hydrochloride (Artane) as an adjunct treatment to levodopa in the management of parkinsonism. To avoid the adverse reactions of Artane, you will teach the client to:

1. take the drug 30 to 45 minutes before meals.
2. consume a high-fiber diet and maintain an adequate fluid intake.
3. void every 2 to 3 hours during the day.
4. have a handkerchief available to cope with drooling.

1 0 - 2 0

An infant is being treated with indomethacin (Indocin) for patent ductus arteriosus (PDA). Which assessment finding should be reported immediately?

1. bleeding from prior heel pricks
2. capillary refill of less than 2 seconds
3. presence of faint murmur that sounds machinery-like, unchanged from previous assessment
4. respiratory rate of 40 breaths per minute and heart rate of 130 beats per minute

Practice Test 10

Answers, Rationales, and Explanations

1 0 - 1

④ **Fluoxetine (Prozac) is used in the treatment of mood disorders. Fluoxetine (Prozac) belongs to a category of drugs called selective serotonin reuptake inhibitors (SSRIs). Because serotonin levels have been found to affect mood, this category of drugs is prescribed to treat mood disorders such as depression.**

1. Digoxin (Lanoxin) is a cardiac glycoside (increases the force of heart contraction) and does not affect mood.

2. Ranitidine (Zantac) is an antiulcer agent and does not affect mood.

3. Atenolol (Tenormin) is an antihypertensive agent and does not affect mood.

Pregnancy Category: B
Client Need: Health Promotion/Maintenance

1 0 - 2

④ **Clients should be monitored for respiratory rate and pattern during the administration of intrathecal morphine since respiratory depression can occur. Morphine sulfate is a narcotic analgesic and may be delivered into the intrathecal space (spinal canal) for a 24-hour duration of action.**

1. Respiratory rates less than 12 are considered reportable.

2. Coughing and deep breathing are encouraged in the postoperative client to prevent pneumonia and atelectasis.

3. Flumazenil (Romazicon) is the agonist (has an affinity for another drug's cellular receptor sites) for benzodiazepines, not narcotic analgesics such as morphine.

Pregnancy Category: C
Client Need: Safe, Effective Care Environment

1 0 - 3

① **Carbidopa-levodopa (Sinemet) replaces dopamine, which is a neurotransmitter. Sinemet is converted to dopamine in the central nervous system (CNS), where it functions as a neurotransmitter.**

2. Carbidopa-levodopa (Sinemet) does not suppress production of dopamine.

3. Carbidopa-levodopa (Sinement) reduces muscle rigidity and tremor. Spasticity is not associated with Parkinson's disease.

4. Carbidopa-levodopa (Sinemet) does not slow nerve impulse transmission. It is a neurotransmitter.

Pregnancy Category: C
Client Need: Psychosocial Integrity

10-4

④ **You will administer an analgesic. The use of analgesics (drugs that relieve pain) should be anticipated during a sickle-cell crisis. Sickle-cell anemia is a hereditary disease in which the red blood cells are sickle-shaped rather than concave dish-shaped. These cells carry oxygen inefficiently and tend to clump, causing ischemia and severe pain.**

1, 2, and 3. Antacids, antiarrhythmics, and antihistamines do not affect pain.

Pregnancy Category: NR
Client Need: Physiological Integrity

10-5

① **Ibuprofen (Motrin) is a nonsteroidal anti-inflammatory drug whose impact on prostaglandin synthesis produces antipyretic and analgesic effects.**

2. Meperidine (Demerol) is a narcotic analgesic.

3. Promethazine (Phenergan) is an antiemetic.

4. Ampicillin (Omnipen) is a penicillin antibiotic.

Pregnancy Category: NR
Client Need: Physiological Integrity

10-6

④ **Morphine sulfate improves circulation and relieves pain. It is a narcotic analgesic (pain reliever). Morphine sulfate increases venous capacity and decreases tension in the heart muscle, which helps circulation to the heart muscle.**

1. Morphine is not a thrombolytic drug (it does not lyse blood clots).

2. Morphine is not a hallucinogenic, although it may produce mild euphoria.

3. Morphine is a central nervous system depressant, not a stimulant.

Pregnancy Category: C
Client Need: Physiological Integrity

10-7

① **Nonsteroidal anti-inflammatory drugs (NSAIDs) increase methotrexate (Rheumatrex) toxicity when used together for pyramid treatment of arthritis.**

2, 3, and 4. There are no known interactions between muscle relaxants, steroidal anti-inflammatory agents, iron supplements, and methotrexate (Rheumatrex).

Pregnancy Category: X
Client Need: Health Promotion/Maintenance

1 0 - 8

① **Clients receiving dopamine (levodopa) should be taught to rise slowly from a sitting position. Orthostatic hypotension is a common side effect of levodopa. Rising slowly to an upright position will prevent dizziness and fainting.**

2. Vitamin B$_6$ tends to reduce the performance of dopamine (levodopa) and should be avoided.

3. Dopamine (levodopa) does cause some sedation. However, restrictions on operating moving vehicles should be determined on an individual basis.

4. Food with high protein content will reduce dopamine's efficacy by diminishing its absorption and should be consumed with this in mind.

Pregnancy Category: C
Client Need: Health Promotion/Maintenance

1 0 - 9

② **Prolonged bleeding is not associated with Tylenol use. However, prolonged bleeding is associated with acute salicylate (aspirin) poisoning. Signs and symptoms of acute poisoning with acetaminophen include: Anorexia, nausea, vomiting, dizziness, lethargy, diaphoresis, chills, epigastric or abdominal pain, diarrhea, hypoglycemia, hepatic coma, and acute renal failure.**

1. The nurse will anticipate the use of acetylcysteine (Mucomyst). Acetylcysteine (Mucomyst) is the antidote for Tylenol overdose. Administered by mouth, it decreases the accumulation of a hepatoxic metabolite found in Tylenol. As an inhalant, it breaks down mucus so that it is less viscous and easier to expectorate.

3. Hypoglycemia may occur with Tylenol overdose and should be monitored.

4. It will be important to monitor liver and renal functions because hepatic necrosis (death of tissue) may occur with Tylenol overdose.

Pregnancy Category: B
Client Need: Physiological Integrity

1 0 - 1 0

② **Ibuprofen (Motrin) is effective in treating tendinitis. Tendinitis is a painful disorder caused by inflammation of the tendon tissue. Ibuprofen is a nonsteroidal anti-inflammatory agent whose analgesic and anti-inflammatory properties make it an effective agent in the treatment of tendinitis.**

1. Acetaminophen (Tylenol) has no anti-inflammatory properties. It is a nonnarcotic analgesic and antipyretic.

3. Liotrix (Euthroid) is a thyroid hormone.

4. Theophylline (Theobid) is a bronchodilator.

Pregnancy Category: NR
Client Need: Physiological Integrity

10-11

1. ① **Analgesics may be prescribed for the pain associated with renal calculi. Renal calculi (kidney stones) are formed from several crystalline sources, including calcium and uric acid. The cardinal sign of this disorder is flank pain (pain located at the side of the body between the ribs and ilium), which is many times described as excruciating. Pain management is one of the priorities in the care of these clients.**

2. Antiarrhythmic medications are not required because there is no indication that the client is experiencing dysrhythmia.

3. Diuretics are prescribed in the management of hypertension or edema associated with conditions such as congestive heart failure. There is no evidence to support the need for diuretics in this situation.

4. Renal calculi are not caused by viruses; therefore, an antiviral agent is not indicated.

Pregnancy Category: NR
Client Need: Physiological Integrity

10-12

1. ① **The client will be instructed to take levodopa (Dopar) with food and before major activities. When taken with food and before activities of the day, levodopa (Dopar) tends to facilitate the client's mobility, minimize GI upset, and promote functional capacity. This occurs because of the medication's impact on neuron conduction.**

2. Levodopa (Dopar) does cause drowsiness. However, it must be taken at frequent intervals during the day to maintain a therapeutic level.

3. Levodopa (Dopar) must be taken on a regular basis in order to maintain a therapeutic level.

4. Levodopa (Dopar) causes gastrointestinal irritation, which can be minimized by taking it with a small amount of food.

Pregnancy Category: C
Client Need: Health Promotion/Maintenance

10-13

1. ① **The nurse should question the dosage of the drug. Fentanyl transdermal (Duragesic) should not be applied daily. Fentanyl transdermal is a narcotic opioid analgesic. The patches are applied every 72 hours. The medication is slowly absorbed into the system and the full analgesic effect is not reached until after 24 hours.**

2. The full analgesic effect of fentanyl transdermal (Duragesic) is not reached until approximately 24 hours after the first application of this medication.

3. Like other opioids, fentanyl transdermal (Duragesic) may cause hypotension and respiratory distress.

4. The application site of fentanyl transdermal (Duragesic) should be alternated in order to avoid irritation of the skin.

Pregnancy Category: C
Client Need: Safe, Effective Care Environment

10-14

① **Divalproex sodium (Depakote) is an anticonvulsant whose impact on neural transmission makes it a very effective drug in the treatment of tonic-clonic seizures (grand mal).**

2. Ranitidine (Zantac) is an antiulcer medication and has no impact on convulsions.

3. Digoxin (Lanoxin) is a cardiac glycoside and has no impact on convulsions.

4. Captopril (Capoten) is an antihypertensive and has no impact on convulsions.

Pregnancy Category: D
Client Need: Physiological Integrity

10-15

③ **Ketorolac (Toradol) is very helpful in relieving the pain associated with fractures. Ketorolac is a nonopioid analgesic, nonsteroidal anti-inflammatory agent whose impact on prostaglandin synthesis makes it very effective.**

1. Furosemide (Lasix) is a loop diuretic and does not provide analgesia.

2. Ranitidine (Zantac) is an antiulcer drug and does not provide analgesia.

4. Bretylium (Bretylol) is an antiarrhythmic and does not provide analgesia.

Pregnancy Category: C
Client Need: Physiological Integrity

10-16

① **A dosage increase of ethinyl estradiol (Estinyl) is anticipated. The hepatic metabolism of ethinyl estradiol (a synthetic estrogen) may be increased by the introduction of Dilantin. The ethinyl estradiol dosage may have to be increased to compensate for this.**

2 and 3. The dosage of ethinyl estradiol will most likely need to be increased.

4. There is no need to anticipate a discontinuation of the ethinyl. Dilantin and ethinyl estradiol can be taken concurrently.

Pregnancy Category: X
Client Need: Health Promotion/Maintenance

10-17

② You will teach clients taking naproxen sodium (Naprelan) that the medication should be taken with food or milk. Naproxen sodium (Naprelan) is a nonsteroidal antiinflammatory (NSAID) used often in the treatment of musculoskeletal injuries. It, like all other NSAIDs, is notoriously ulcerogenic and must be taken with food or milk to prevent gastrointestinal distress.

1. Naproxen sodium (Naprelan) is a nonsteroidal anti-inflammatory medication (NSAID), not a narcotic.

3. Naproxen sodium (Naprelan) is contraindicated for clients with peptic ulcer disease because of its ulcerogenic properties.

4. Naproxen sodium (Naprelan) must be taken with food because of its irritating effects on the gastrointestinal mucosa.

Pregnancy Category: B
Client Need: Physiological Integrity

10-18

③ You will anticipate a prescription for chlordiazepoxide hydrochloride (Librium). Librium is an antianxiety drug that is effective in treating mild to severe anxiety. Clients experiencing delirium tremens (DTs) are likely to experience anxiety in association with delusions and hallucinations.

1. Stelazine is an antipsychotic agent normally administered to clients diagnosed with schizophrenia or other psychotic disorders.

2. Disulfiram (Antabuse) is an antagonist which, when combined with alcohol consumption, produces unpleasant effects such as: Flushing, throbbing headache, dyspnea, nausea, vomiting, diaphoresis, palpitations, and anxiety. It is hoped that these unpleasant adverse reactions will influence alcoholics not to drink when taking Antabuse.

4. Fluphenazine enanthate (Prolixin) is an antipsychotic agent normally administered to treat psychotic disorders.

Pregnancy Category: NR
Client Need: Physiological Integrity

1 0 - 1 9

② **You will teach your client to consume a high-fiber diet and maintain an adequate fluid intake due to the potential for constipation and dry mouth associated with the administration of trihexyphenidyl hydrochloride (Artane).**

1.   Adverse reactions to trihexyphenidyl hydrochloride (Artane) include: Nausea, vomiting, dry mouth, constipation, and urinary hesitancy/retention. Taking Artane 30 to 40 minutes before meals will not prevent these adverse reactions.

3.   Urinary hesitancy/retention is an adverse reaction to the drug trihexyphenidyl hydrochloride (Artane). Treating these conditions includes voiding when the urge occurs, which may or may not be every 2 to 3 hours.

4.   The administration of trihexyphenidyl hydrochloride (Artane) is associated with dry mouth, not drooling. A handkerchief should not be necessary.

Pregnancy Category: NR

Client Need: Health Promotion/Maintenance

1 0 - 2 0

① **Bleeding from prior heel prick sites should be reported to the physician immediately. Indomethacin is a nonsteroidal anti-inflammatory used as an alternative to surgery for clients with patent ductus arteriosus. Indomethacin inhibits platelet function; therefore, the nurse should observe for bleeding.**

2.   Capillary refill of less than 2 seconds indicates good peripheral perfusion and low probability of congestive heart failure.

3.   The presence of a faint machinery-like murmur is typical of patent ductus arteriosus (PDA).

4.   A respiratory rate of 40 breaths per minute is within normal limits (30 to 50) for an infant. A heart rate of 130 beats per minute (BPM) is within normal limits (120 to 160) for an infant.

Pregnancy Category: NR

Client Need: Physiological Integrity

Practice Test 11

Nutritional Agents

OVERVIEW

Nutritional agents treat, prevent, and inhibit various vitamin and mineral deficiencies. They are also administered as supplements in metabolic disorders.

Nutritional agents include:

- Calories
- Minerals
- Vitamins

CALORIES

A calorie is a unit of heat. In connection with nutrition, calories (Kilocalories) refer to the energy content of food (that is, the fuel or energy value of the food).

Conditions treated with calories include:

- Anorexia
- Marasmic kwashiorkor (severe calorie and protein deficiency)

MINERALS

Minerals are inorganic elements or compounds occurring in nature. Minerals are necessary constituents of all body cells. They form the largest part of the hard portions of the body, such as bone, nails, and teeth. Minerals regulate the permeability of cell membranes and capillaries, the excitability of muscle and nerve tissue, osmotic pressure, equilibrium, acid-base balance, and blood volume. They are also constituents of secretions from glands. Some of the principal minerals include: Calcium, iodine, phosphorus, potassium, and sodium.

Conditions treated with minerals include:

- Muscle cramps (treated with sodium)
- Muscle weakness, changes in electrocardiogram (treated with potassium)
- Retarded growth, weakness (treated with phosphorus)
- Rickets, tetany, brittle bones (treated with calcium)
- Simple goiter (treated with iodine)

VITAMINS

Vitamins are essential for normal growth and good nutrition. Most vitamins are acquired from outside sources, such as food, because they cannot be manufactured by the body. There are vitamins, however, that can be manufactured by the body; they are vitamins A and K. Vitamins are found in two main groupings: the water-soluble vitamins (vitamin C and the B complex vitamins B_1, B_2, B_3, B_5, B_6, B_{12}) and the fat-soluble vitamins (vitamins A, D, E, K).

Conditions treated with water-soluble vitamins include:

- Anemia (treated with vitamin B_{12})
- Beriberi (treated with vitamin B)
- Scurvy (treated with vitamin C)
- Wounds (treated with vitamin C)

Conditions treated with fat-soluble vitamins include:

- Hypoprothrombinemia (lack of blood-clotting Factor II, treated with vitamin K)
- Night blindness (treated with vitamin A)
- Rickets/osteomalacia (treated with vitamin D)

Practice Test 11

Questions

11-1

Your 52-year-old client is concerned about the potential effects of osteoporosis. The client has increased dietary intake of calcium. You will teach the client that the absorption of calcium is enhanced by the ingestion of:

1. vitamin C.
2. vitamin A.
3. vitamin D.
4. vitamin B.

11-2

A client states, "My stools have been really dark lately." Which of the following medications has probably caused this change?

1. ferrous sulfate
2. calcium carbonate
3. Ranitidine
4. folic acid

11-3

How might parenteral iron dextran be administered?

1. subcutaneously
2. by rapid intravenous bolus
3. intradermally
4. intramuscularly

11-4

You are to administer pancrelipase (Pancrease) to a child with pancreatic insufficiency. Your teaching about this medication will include:

1. Hypouricemia can result from the use of this enzyme.
2. Pancrelipase is activated by acids.
3. Tablets should not be chewed.
4. Enzyme activity is decreased if the medication is taken along with histamine (H_2) receptor antagonists.

1 1 - 5

Which of the following will be prescribed for a client diagnosed with pernicious anemia?

1. vitamin B_3
2. vitamin C
3. vitamin A
4. vitamin B_{12}

1 1 - 6

One of the first detectable signs of vitamin A deficiency is:

1. beriberi.
2. pellagra.
3. scurvy.
4. night blindness.

1 1 - 7

Your client is taking a calcium supplement to treat hypocalcemia. To facilitate absorption and utilization of the supplement, you will teach the client to consume foods high in:

1. phosphorus.
2. magnesium.
3. vitamin D.
4. vitamin B_1.

1 1 - 8

A client with hepatitis is experiencing bleeding tendencies. You understand that these tendencies are caused by the lack of:

1. vitamin C.
2. vitamin A.
3. vitamin K.
4. vitamin B.

1 1 - 9

To promote tissue repair, you will encourage your client to consume foods high in vitamin A, such as:

1. sweet potatoes.
2. peanuts.
3. kidney beans.
4. oatmeal.

11-10

You understand that clients with pernicious anemia will require lifelong monthly injections of:

1. cholecalciferol.
2. ascorbic acid.
3. cyanocobalamin.
4. thiamine hydrochloride.

11-11

Your client has osteoporosis. To treat this condition, you will teach the client to consume foods from which of the following groups?

1. milk products
2. meats
3. vegetables
4. fruits

11-12

Your client had a cholecystectomy. To promote tissue repair, you will encourage foods high in vitamin:

1. A.
2. B_6.
3. C.
4. D.

11-13

Which of the following vitamins depresses the synthesis of fatty acids?

1. vitamin B_3
2. vitamin A
3. vitamin C
4. vitamin K

11-14

An infant has been diagnosed with kwashiorkor. Which of the following food deficiencies best describes this condition?

1. protein-calorie malnutrition
2. protein deficiency regardless of adequate calories
3. vitamin A deficiency
4. vitamin B_1 deficiency

1 1 - 1 5

A client has been diagnosed with hyperthyroidism and thyroid hypertrophy. Which of the following best describes this condition?

1. hypervitaminoses A and D
2. protein-calorie malnutrition
3. low serum levels of zinc
4. insufficient intake of dietary iodine

1 1 - 1 6

Vitamin E deficiency is best described as a:

1. deficit of the element necessary for the formation of prothrombin and other clotting factors.
2. deficit causing anorexia, weight loss, abdominal discomfort, sore mouth, diarrhea, and constipation.
3. deficit that interferes with normal bone calcification.
4. deficit that manifests as hemolytic anemia.

Practice Test 11

Answers, Rationales, and Explanations

11 - 1

③ **You will teach the client that calcium absorption is enhanced by ingestion of vitamin D. Vitamin D is a fat-soluble vitamin. A deficiency of vitamin D inhibits the absorption of calcium. Osteoporosis can be treated with increased amounts of calcium and vitamin D.**

1. Vitamin C enhances the absorption of iron.

2. A deficiency of vitamin A causes xerophthalmia (a disease of the eyes that causes blindness).

4. A deficiency in vitamin B complex (including B_1, B_2, B_6, B_{12}) causes the disease beriberi.

Pregnancy Category: C
Client Need: Health Promotion/Maintenance

11 - 2

① **Ferrous sulfate (Fer-Iron) has caused the change. The iron salts present in oral ferrous sulfate are excreted into the stool, giving them a dark color. To prevent undue anxiety, clients should be informed that their stools are likely to be dark in color.**

2. Calcium carbonate (Tums) will not cause stools to become dark in color. However, severe constipation may indicate Tums toxicity.

3. Ranitidine (Zantac) does not cause stools to become dark in color.

4. Folic acid (vitamin B_9) may cause urine to be a bright yellow but does not cause stools to become dark in color.

Pregnancy Category: A
Client Need: Physiological Integrity

11 - 3

④ **Iron dextran (InFeD) should be given intramuscularly. Because iron dextran is very irritating and can stain the skin, it is usually given deep and in a large muscle (intramuscularly) using the Z-track technique. To help with absorption, the injection site should be massaged.**

1. Iron is irritating and should not be given subcutaneously. It is thick and may cause an abscess in superficial tissue.

2. When iron is administered intravenously, it should be infused slowly, not as a bolus.

3. Iron should not be given intradermally. Deep intramuscular injections are required to prevent abcesses and staining of skin and to facilitate absorption.

1 1 - 4

③ **Capsules and tablets of pancrelipase (Pancrease) should not be chewed. Chewing the capsules or tablets exposes the enzyme to gastric acid. Pancrelipase is inactivated by an acidic environment. Enteric-coated capsules or tablets (microspheres or microtablets) delay the activation of the enzyme until the medication has reached the duodenum. Cimetidine, ranitidine, or an antacid may be prescribed to be taken before pancrelipase to prevent destruction of the pancrelipase by gastric pepsin and acid pH.**

1. Hyperuricemia (an excess of uric acid or urates in the blood) may result from the use of pancrelipase (Pancrease).
2. Pancrelipase is inactivated by acids; therefore, tablets and capsules should not be chewed.
4. Enzyme activity is increased if taken along with histamine (H_2) receptor antagonists.

Pregnancy Category: C

Client Need: Health Promotion/Maintenance

1 1 - 5

④ **The nurse will anticipate a prescription for vitamin B_{12} for clients with pernicious anemia. Pernicious anemia is a low red blood cell count due to bone marrow changes as a result of low vitamin B_{12} levels. Vitamin B_{12} is necessary for the synthesis of red blood cells.**

1. Vitamin B_3 has no impact on bone marrow and the management of pernicious anemia. It is used to treat and prevent pellagra and hyperlipidemia.
2. Vitamin C has no impact on bone marrow and the management of pernicious anemia. Its uses include the treatment and prevention of scurvy.
3. Vitamin A has no impact on bone marrow and the management of pernicious anemia. Its uses include the treatment of acne and maintenance of retinal function.

Pregnancy Category: C

Client Need: Physiological Integrity

1 1 - 6

④ **Night blindness is one of the first detectable signs of vitamin A deficiency.**

1. Beriberi is a condition caused by the lack of vitamin B (thiamine). Early deficiency causes fatigue, poor memory, anorexia, and sleep disturbance.
2. Pellagra is a condition caused by the lack of niacin. Symptoms of pellagra include: Dermatitis, inflammation of the mucous membranes, diarrhea, and mental disturbance.
3. Scurvy is caused by the lack of vitamin C. Symptoms of scurvy include: Weakness, anemia, and spongy gums.

Pregnancy Category: C

Client Need: Physiological Integrity

1 1 - 7

③ **You will teach the client to consume foods high in vitamin D. Vitamin D facilitates the absorption and utilization of calcium. Sources of vitamin D include: Egg yolks, milk, and salmon.**

1. Phosphorus is a mineral. It does not facilitate the absorption of calcium; in fact, an excess of phosphorus may pull calcium out of the body.

2. Magnesium is involved in bone mineralization. However, it does not facilitate the absorption of calcium.

4. The chief functions of vitamin B_1 include support of normal appetite and nervous system function. It does not facilitate the absorption of calcium.

Pregnancy Category: C
Client Need: Health Promotion/Maintenance

1 1 - 8

③ **You understand that bleeding tendencies are due to a lack of vitamin K. Vitamin K is a fat-soluble vitamin. Clients who have hepatitis have a decrease in vitamin K absorption due to a reduction of bile in the intestine.**

1. Adequate amounts of vitamin C (ascorbic acid) are required to maintain the integrity of blood vessels. Without adequate vitamin C, bleeding tendencies may occur. However, hepatitis does not affect the absorption of vitamin C.

2. Conditions associated with vitamin A deficiency include: Night blindness and hyperkeratosis (overgrowth of the horny layer of the epidermis), not bleeding tendencies.

4. Conditions associated with vitamin B deficiency include: Beriberi and pellagra, not bleeding tendencies.

Pregnancy Category: A
Client Need: Physiological Integrity

1 1 - 9

① **Sweet potatoes are high in vitamin A. Beef liver, carrots, spinach, squash, and dandelion greens are also high in vitamin A.**

2. Peanuts have very little vitamin A.

3. Kidney beans are not a source of vitamin A.

4. Oatmeal is not high in vitamin A.

Pregnancy Category: C
Client Need: Health Promotion/Maintenance

11-10

③ **Cyanocobalamin (vitamin B$_{12}$) injections are required monthly on a lifelong basis for clients with pernicious anemia. Iron and diet are also included in the treatment plan. Pernicious anemia occurs due to a failure of the stomach to secrete enough intrinsic factor to ensure intestinal absorption of cyanocobalamin (Vitamin B$_{12}$).**

1. Cholecalciferol (vitamin D) may be administered to treat rickets, not pernicious anemia.
2. Ascorbic acid (vitamin C) may be administered to treat scurvy, not pernicious anemia.
4. Thiamine hydrochloride (vitamin B$_1$) may be given to treat beriberi, not pernicious anemia.

Pregnancy Category: C (if used in doses above the RDA)
Client Need: Health Promotion/Maintenance

11-11

① **You will teach your client that milk products are high in calcium. Two or more selections from the milk group help to meet the USDA-recommended daily allowance (RDA) for calcium intake. Osteoporosis is a reduction in the mass of bone per unit of volume. The bones most frequently involved are the vertebrae of the lower dorsal and lumbar areas.**

2. Meats are not a high source of calcium. Meats are usually consumed for their high protein content.
3. Some vegetables, such as spinach, turnips, and broccoli, are good sources of calcium, but they are not as high in calcium as milk and milk products.
4. Fruits are not a good source of calcium.

Pregnancy Category: NA
Client Need: Health Promotion/Maintenance

11-12

① **Vitamin A is associated with tissue repair, good night vision, and maintenance of healthy mucous membranes and skin. Foods high in vitamin A include: Sweet potatoes, carrots, spinach, and squash.**

2. The chief function of vitamin B$_6$ includes: The promotion of new cell synthesis.
3. The chief functions of vitamin C include: Strengthening blood vessels, formation of scar tissue, resistance to infection, and absorption of iron.
4. Vitamin K is necessary for the clotting of blood.

Pregnancy Category: C
Client Need: Physiological Integrity

11-13

① Vitamin B$_3$ depresses the synthesis of fatty acids. Vitamin B$_3$ (also known as niacin or nicotinic acid) is an antilipemic. It directly stimulates the metabolism of lipids and depresses the synthesis of other fatty proteins. Meat, poultry, and fish are the sources of approximately 50% of the niacin consumed by Americans. Other sources high in niacin include enriched breads and cereals. Green leafy vegetables are also rich sources of niacin.

2. Vitamin A is a fat-soluble vitamin that promotes good night vision, healthy mucous membranes and skin, and the growth of body tissues. It is not an antilipemic.

3. Vitamin C is an antioxidant necessary in maintaining the integrity of blood vessels. An inadequate amount of vitamin C causes scurvy. Fruits and vegetables supply rich amounts of vitamin C. Vitamin C is not an antilipemic.

4. Vitamin K acts primarily in the clotting of blood. Significant sources of vitamin K are: Liver, green leafy vegetables, and milk. Vitamin K is not an antilipemic.

Pregnancy Category: C
Client Need: Physiological Integrity

11-14

② Kwashiorkor results from protein deficiency regardless of adequate calories. Children with kwashiorkor may be lethargic, irritable, and anorexic. Growth retardation can be less pronounced than in marasmus (general wasting away of infants due to malnutrition). Treatment involves high-quality protein foods and protein caloric supplements.

1. Protein-calorie malnutrition is referred to as marasmus. Infants with marasmus experience growth retardation, emaciation, physical inactivity, apathy, frequent infections, anorexia, weakness, irritability, hunger, diarrhea, and nausea and vomiting.

3. Vitamin A deficiency refers to inadequate dietary intake of foods high in vitamin A, such as carrots, sweet potatoes, and squash. Vitamin A maintains epithelial tissue and retinal function. Lack of vitamin A causes night blindness and dry, scaly skin. Where there is corneal damage, emergency treatment is required.

4. Vitamin B$_1$ deficiency refers to malabsorption or inadequate dietary intake of thiamine. Early complaints include anorexia, irritability, muscle cramps, and paresthesia (a tingling sensation); advanced deficiency is associated with heart and nervous system disease.

Pregnancy Category: NR
Client Need: Health Promotion/Maintenance

11-15

④ **Hyperthyroidism and thyroid hypertrophy (endemic goiter) can result from iodine deficiency. Other effects range from dental caries to cretinism (mental retardation) in infants. Treatment consists of iodine supplements.**

1. Hypervitaminoses A and D refers to the accumulation of excessive amounts of vitamin A and D. The accumulation occurs because these vitamins are not dissolved and excreted in the urine.

2. Protein-calorie malnutrition is referred to as marasmus. Kwashiorkor is protein deficiency despite adequate calorie intake.

3. A low serum level of zinc occurs when there is excessive intake of foods that bind to zinc and take it out of the body. Other causes of low serum zinc levels include malabsorption disorders and malnutrition, resulting in sparse hair growth, soft, misshapen nails, and dry, scaly skin. Treatment is correcting the underlying cause and administering supplements.

Pregnancy Category: C
Client Need: Health Promotion/Maintenance

11-16

④ **Vitamin E deficiency manifests as hemolytic anemia in low birth weight or premature infants. Vitamin E deficiency among infants commonly occurs from feeding with formulas high in polyunsaturated fatty acids that are fortified with iron but not vitamin E. Hemolytic anemia also develops in conditions associated with fat malabsorption. Signs and symptoms include edema and skin lesions. Adults may have muscle weakness, intermittent claudication, and joint disturbances. Treatment: Replacement of vitamin E with supplements.**

1. A vitamin K deficiency is best described as a deficit of the element necessary for the formation of prothrombin and other clotting factors. Treatment: Vitamin K with monitoring of prothrombin time.

2. A vitamin B_{12} (cyanocobalamin) deficiency is best described as a deficit causing anorexia, weight loss, abdominal discomfort, sore mouth, diarrhea, and constipation.

3. A vitamin D deficiency is best described as a deficit that interferes with bone calcification.

Pregnancy Category: A
Client Need: Physiological Integrity

Practice Test 12

Ophthalmic, Otic, and Nasal Agents

OVERVIEW

Ophthalmic, otic, and nasal agents treat, prevent, and inhibit conditions affecting the eyes, ears, and nose.

Ophthalmic, otic, and nasal agents include:

- Miotics
- Mydriatics
- Nasal agents
- Ophthalmic anti-infectives
- Ophthalmic anti-inflammatories
- Ophthalmic vasoconstrictors
- Otics

MIOTICS

Miotics cause the pupil to contract (constrict).

Miotic substances include:

- Carbachol (intraocular) (Miostat)
- Pilocarpine (Piloptic)

Conditions treated with miotics include:

- Primary open-angle glaucoma
- Miotics are also administered to create pupillary miosis (contraction) in ocular surgery.

MYDRIATICS

Mydriatics dilate the pupil. In certain diseases of the eye, the pupil must be dilated during treatment to prevent adhesions of the pupils.

Mydriatics include:

- Atropine sulfate (Atropine-1)
- Cyclopentolate hydrochloride (Mydrilate)
- Epinephrine hydrochloride (Glaucon)

Conditions treated with mydriatics include:

- Cycloplegia (paralysis of ciliary muscles)
- Open-angle glaucoma

NASAL AGENTS

Nasal agents are administered to treat various conditions of the nose.

Nasal agents include:

- Beclomethasone dipropionate (Beconase)
- Fluticasone propionate (Flonase)
- Oxymetazoline hydrochloride (Afrin)
- Phenylephrine hydrochloride (Neo-Synephrine)

Conditions treated with nasal agents include:

- Nasal congestion
- Nosebleed
- Seasonal and perennial allergic rhinitis

OPHTHALMIC ANTI-INFECTIVES

Ophthalmic anti-infectives are administered to treat or prevent infections in the eyes.

Ophthalmic anti-infectives include:

- Bacitracin (AK-Tracin)
- Erythromycin ointment
- Silver nitrate solution

Conditions treated with ophthalmic anti-infectives include:

- Conjunctivitis
- Corneal ulcers
- Corneitis
- Ophthalmia neonatorum, as prophylaxis

OPHTHALMIC ANTI-INFLAMMATORIES

Ophthalmic anti-inflammatories are administered to treat tissue reactions to various types of injury to the eyes caused by surgery, allergy, and foreign objects.

Ophthalmic anti-inflammatories include:

- Dexamethasone (Maxidex)
- Diclofenac sodium (Voltaren Ophthalmic)
- Fluorometholone (Flarex)

Conditions treated with ophthalmic anti-inflammatories include:

- Corneal injury from burns, chemicals, and penetration of foreign objects
- Inflammatory allergic conditions of conjunctiva, cornea, and sclera
- Inflammatory conditions of the eyelids
- Postoperative inflammation following removal of a cataract

OPHTHALMIC VASOCONSTRICTORS

Ophthalmic vasoconstrictors constrict blood vessels and the pupil of the eye.

Ophthalmic vasoconstrictors include:

- Naphazoline hydrochloride (Allerest)
- Oxymetazoline hydrochloride (Visine)
- Tetrahydrozoline hydrochloride (Collyrium)

Conditions treated with ophthalmic vasoconstrictors include:

- Allergies
- Minor eye irritations
- Ocular congestion, irritation, itching

OTICS

Otics are administered to treat various conditions of the ear.

Otics include:

- Boric acid solution (Ear-dry)
- Carbamide peroxide (Murine Ear)

Conditions treated with otics include:

- External ear canal infection
- Impacted cerumen (earwax)

Practice Test 12

Questions

1 2 - 1

The nurse administers tetracycline ointment rather than silver nitrate for a newborn's prophylactic eye care. Silver nitrate is used less frequently because it:

1. causes brown staining of the skin it touches.
2. does not prevent chlamydial infection.
3. is more difficult to administer.
4. must be rinsed from the eye after 1 minute.

1 2 - 2

A client with asthma talks to you about the medications she is taking. Which drug would be contraindicated?

1. nystatin (Mycostatin) vaginal inserts
2. desoximetasone (Topicort) ointment
3. pilocarpine (Carpine) ophthalmic solution
4. nitroglycerin (Transderm-Nitro) 2 mg/24-hour patch

1 2 - 3

A client with seasonal rhinitis is to receive beclomethasone dipropionate (Beconase). The drug will be sprayed in each nostril tid. To administer this drug, you will teach the client to:

1. tilt the head slightly backward and insert the nozzle into the nostril.
2. rotate the medication gently between the palms of the hands prior to administration.
3. blow the nose to clear the nasal passages prior to administration.
4. keep both nostrils open while instilling the medication.

1 2 - 4

A client is seen in the Emergency Department following accidental trauma to the nose. To treat the superficial bleeding of the client's nasal membranes, you anticipate a prescription for:

1. flunisolide (Nasalide).
2. epinephrine hydrochloride (Adrenalin Chloride).
3. fluticasone propionate (Flonase).
4. triamcinolone acetonide (Nasacort).

1 2 - 5

You are to administer carbamide peroxide (Murine Ear) to treat impacted cerumen. You know to:

1. instill 5 to 10 drops into the ear canal.
2. instill the drops daily for up to 7 days.
3. allow the drops to remain in the ears for several hours.
4. remove the dissolved cerumen with cool water.

1 2 - 6

A client with acquired immunodeficiency syndrome (AIDS) has contracted an opportunistic infection of the eyes (cytomegalovirus/CMV). You anticipate the administration of ganciclovir (Cytovene). You will teach the client that this drug:

1. causes birth defects.
2. may be administered as an intravenous bolus.
3. may be given initially q 12 hours for 7 to 14 days.
4. is unlikely to cause nausea or vomiting.

1 2 - 7

Your client is scheduled for an intracapsular cataract extraction (ICCE) and is to receive an intravenous injection of methohexital sodium (Brevital). You know the purpose of this medication is to:

1. provide a prophylactic against infection following surgery.
2. dilate the client's pupils.
3. reduce intraocular pressure.
4. provide a few minutes of light anesthesia.

1 2 - 8

It has become necessary to schedule a mastoidectomy for a client experiencing chronic otitis media. Postoperative nursing actions will include the use of hydrogen peroxide solution for postauricular care. You know the primary purpose of this drug is to:

1. kill bacteria at the postoperative site.
2. soften the tissue at the suture site.
3. cleanse the postoperative site.
4. minimize the potential for infection.

1 2 - 9

A client has bilateral nasal polyps. To temporarily reduce the polyps, you anticipate a prescription for:

1. corticosteroids.
2. antihistamines.
3. anti-infectives.
4. astringents.

Practice Test 12

Answers, Rationales, and Explanations

1 2 - 1

②   **Silver nitrate is not usually administered for a newborn's prophylactic eye care because it does not prevent chlamydial infection. Silver nitrate prevents only ophthalmia neonatorum (acute purulent conjunctivitis) caused by the gonococcus. Tetracycline and erythromycin prevent ophthalmia neonatorum and chlamydia.**

1.   Silver nitrate does not prevent chlamydial infection. It does cause brown staining of the skin it touches, but this is only temporary.

3.   Silver nitrate is no more difficult to administer than tetracycline and erythromycin. Tetracycline is administered as a thin strip ointment or as a one-drop suspension for prophylactic eye care in the newborn. Erythromycin is administered as a thin strip ointment for prophylactic eye care in the newborn.

4.   The eye should not be irrigated after instillation of silver nitrate drops. Excess silver nitrate should be wiped from eyelids and surrounding skin.

Pregnancy Category: C

Client Need: Health Promotion/Maintenance

1 2 - 2

③   **Pilocarpine (Carpine) ophthalmic solution is contraindicated for clients with asthma. Pilocarpine is a miotic solution (causes pupils to contract) used in the treatment of glaucoma. It is a cholinergic that is systemically absorbed and may cause bronchospasm or bronchoconstriction.**

1.   Nystatin (Mycostatin) vaginal inserts do not cause bronchospasm or bronchoconstriction and are not contraindicated for clients with asthma. This medication is administered for the treatment of local and intestinal candida infections.

2.   Desoximetasone (Topicort) ointment does not cause bronchospasm or bronchoconstriction and is not contraindicated for clients with asthma. This medication is a topical glucocorticoid used to manage a variety of allergic immunologic reactions.

4.   Nitroglycerin (Transderm-Nitro) is used in the long-term prophylactic management of angina pectoris. It does not cause bronchospasm or bronchoconstriction.

Pregnancy Category: B

Client Need: Safe, Effective Care Environment

1 2 - 3

③   **The client will be taught to blow the nose and clear the nasal passages to ensure that the medication can be absorbed properly; otherwise, the medication will not come in contact with the mucous membranes of the nose and be absorbed into the bloodstream.**

1.   The client should tilt the head slightly forward to insert the nozzle into the nostril. This technique allows the medication to adhere to the nasal membranes as opposed to having the medication become lost down the throat when the head is tilted backward.

2.   The container should be shaken well before use. This technique allows the suspension to be evenly distributed when sprayed.

4.   When instilling spray into a nostril, the other nostril should be closed. The client should inspire gently when spraying medication into the nose.

Pregnancy Category: C

Client Need: Physiological Integrity

1 2 - 4

② **You will anticipate a prescription for epinephrine hydrochloride (Adrenalin Chloride). This medication causes local vasoconstriction of dilated arterioles, which in turn reduces blood flow. It is administered as a 0.1% nasal solution.**

1. Flunisolide (Nasalide) is a nasal inhalant administered to treat symptoms of seasonal or perennial rhinitis. One of the many adverse reactions is epistaxis (nosebleed).

3. Fluticasone propionate (Flonase) is a nasal spray administered to treat seasonal and perennial allergic rhinitis. An adverse reaction is epistaxis (nosebleed).

4. Triamcinolone acetonide (Nasacort) is a nasal spray pump given to treat and relieve symptoms of seasonal and perennial allergic rhinitis. Adverse reactions include epistaxis (nosebleed).

Pregnancy Category: C
Client Need: Physiological Integrity

1 2 - 5

① **You will instill 5 to 10 drops of carbamide peroxide (Murine Ear) into each of the client's ears. This medication is a ceruminolytic (an agent that dissolves cerumen/earwax in the external ear canals).**

2. You will instill carbamide peroxide (Murine Ear) eardrops for up to 4 days. It should not take more than 4 days of administration to dissolve cerumen (earwax).

3. The solution of carbamide peroxide (Murine Ear) should remain in the external ear canals for several minutes. This will allow sufficient time for the drops to dissolve the cerumen (earwax).

4. The water used to flush out the ear canals should be warm. Warm water will maintain the dissolved cerumen at a consistency that will be easy to remove.

Pregnancy Category: NR
Client Need: Health Promotion/Maintenance

1 2 - 6

① **Ganciclovir (Cytovene) causes birth defects. Female clients taking this drug should be taught to use effective birth control methods during treatment. Male clients should be taught to use barrier contraception during therapy and for a minimum of 90 days following treatment.**

2. Ganciclovir (Cytovene) should not be given as an intravenous bolus. It should be administered over a minimum of 1 hour. Infusions that are too rapid may result in increased toxicity. An infusion pump should be used.

3. The client receiving ganciclovir (Cytovene) normally receives 5 mg/kg intravenously every 12 hours for 14 to 21 days initially.

4. Nausea, vomiting, diarrhea, anorexia, abdominal discomfort, flatulence, and dyspepsia are common adverse reactions to ganciclovir (Cytovene).

Pregnancy Category: C
Client Need: Physiological Integrity

1 2 - 7

④ **Methohexital (Brevital) provides a light anesthesia over a brief period of time. Prior to cataract removal, the drug is administered as an intravenous injection to offer anesthesia while a local anesthetic is injected directly behind the eyeball.**

1. Methohexital (Brevital) is not an anti-infective and would have no effect against the potential for infection following surgery.

2. Methohexital (Brevital) provides a light anesthesia. It does not have mydriatic effects (dilation of pupils).

3. Methohexital (Brevital) does not reduce intraocular pressure. It is a short-acting anesthetic.

Pregnancy Category: C
Client Need: Health Promotion/Maintenance

1 2 - 8

④ **Hydrogen peroxide used in this situation will minimize the potential for infection. Hydrogen peroxide can kill bacteria, and it is also an excellent cleansing agent that loosens adherent deposits and detritus (degenerative matter). It prevents postoperative infection to the auricula by keeping the suture site clean.**

1. Hydrogen peroxide can kill bacteria (it is a germicidal). However, in this situation its purpose is to minimize infection by maintaining a clean postoperative site.

2. Hydrogen peroxide is not a lubricant and will not soften the tissue at the suture site.

3. Hydrogen peroxide can keep the postoperative site clean. However, the ultimate purpose for keeping the site clean is to minimize the potential for infection.

Pregnancy Category: Not Known
Client Need: Health Promotion/Maintenance

1 2 - 9

① **You will anticipate a prescription for corticosteroids. Corticosteroids can be administered by direct injection into the polyps (benign edematous growths) or by local spray. This will physically reduce the polyps.**

2. Antihistamines may be prescribed to control allergy but not to physically reduce the polyps.

3. Anti-infectives would not be anticipated unless there was evidence to suggest an infection.

4. Astringents may be administered for the purpose of shrinking hypertrophied tissues, not polyps.

Pregnancy Category: C
Client Need: Physiological Integrity

Practice Test 13

Respiratory Tract Agents

OVERVIEW

Respiratory tract agents treat, prevent, and inhibit conditions associated with ventilation, perfusion, and diffusion that interfere with the interchange of gases between clients and the air they breathe.

Respiratory tract agents include:

- Antihistamines
- Antitussives
- Bronchodilators
- Mucolytics and expectorants

ANTIHISTAMINES

Histamine is present in various tissues of the body. Histamine acts on the vascular system by producing dilation of the arterioles and increased permeability of capillaries and venules. Antihistamines are administered to counteract the effects of histamine. Antihistamines block almost all the effects of histamine by competing with it at the histamine receptor sites. Antihistamines constrict vessels.

Antihistamines include:

- Cetirizine hydrochloride (Zyrtec)
- Clemastine fumarate (Tavist)
- Diphenhydramine hydrochloride (Benadryl)

Conditions treated with antihistamines include:

- Chronic idiopathic urticaria
- Motion sickness
- Seasonal allergic rhinitis

ANTITUSSIVES

Antitussives are used to relieve coughing. CENTRALLY ACTING ANTITUSSIVES depress the cough center located in the medulla. PERIPHERALLY ACTING ANTITUSSIVES anesthetize receptors in the respiratory passages.

Centrally acting antitussives include:

- Codeine
- Dextromethorphan

Peripherally acting antitussives include:

- Benzonatate (Tessalon)

Conditions treated with antitussives include:

- Nonproductive cough
- Coughing, for symptomatic relief

BRONCHODILATORS

Bronchodilators dilate (open) the bronchus. There are two divisions of bronchodilators:

(1) Sympathomimetics, which dilate the bronchus by their beta-adrenergic activity.

(2) Xanthine derivatives, which dilate the bronchus by directly relaxing the smooth muscle of the bronchus.

Sympathomimetic bronchodilators include:

- Albuterol (Ventolin)
- Terbutaline (Bricanyl)

Xanthine-derivative bronchodilators include:

- Aminophylline (Truphylline)
- Epinephrine hydrochloride (Adrenalin Chloride)
- Theophylline (Theolair liquid)

Conditions treated with bronchodilators include:

- Anaphylaxis
- Bronchial asthma
- Bronchospasm

MUCOLYTICS AND EXPECTORANTS

MUCOLYTICS loosen secretions in the respiratory tract. EXPECTORANTS assist the client in coughing up thick, tenacious mucus from the respiratory tract.

Mucolytics include:

- Acetylcysteine (Mucomyst)

Expectorants include:

- Guaifenesin (Robitussin)

Conditions treated with mucolytics and expectorants include:

- Thick secretions in clients with pneumonia, as adjunct therapy
- Chronic asthma
- Cough due to cold or minor bronchial irritation
- Respiratory conditions associated with dry, unproductive cough

Practice Test 13

Questions

1 3 - 1

A client states, "Before I came today I used my Primatene Mist inhaler." The nurse will anticipate which of the following assessment findings?

1. hypotension
2. bradycardia
3. drowsiness
4. tachycardia

1 3 - 2

Your client, a steroid-dependent asthmatic, has begun a regimen that includes a beclomethasone (Beclovent) inhaler. You will teach the client to:

1. use the inhaler when an asthmatic attack begins.
2. keep the inhaler refrigerated at all times.
3. adjust the number of puffs daily as needed.
4. rinse the mouth well after each use.

1 3 - 3

A client tells you, "Recently my pulse has been racing and I am having difficulty sleeping." Which of the following medications would most likely cause these symptoms?

1. metoprolol (Lopressor)
2. alprazolam (Xanax)
3. aspirin (acetylsalicylic acid)
4. terbutaline (Brethine)

1 3 - 4

Which of the following medications is a bronchodilator and may be prescribed, along with other medications, to treat pneumococcal pneumonia?

1. albuterol (Ventolin)
2. beclomethasone (Vanceril)
3. ampicillin (Omnipen)
4. acetaminophen (Tylenol)

1 3 - 5

Your client is receiving a continuous aminophylline (Palaron) drip. Aminophylline affects the heart by:

1. strengthening the heartbeat.
2. increasing the heart rate.
3. dilating coronary arteries.
4. decreasing myocardial oxygen demand.

1 3 - 6

A client is brought to the Emergency Department after consuming an evening meal. The client's tongue is swelling and obstructing the airway. The most appropriate therapy would be:

1. oxygen via nasal cannula at 2 L/min.
2. oxygen via humified facemask at 100%.
3. oxygen via bag-valve mask at 100%.
4. oxygen via emergency tracheostomy at 100%.

1 3 - 7

A client is apneic as a consequence of anaphylactic shock. Which is the most appropriate treatment?

1. intubation and 100% oxygen
2. diphenhydramine (Benadryl)
3. acetaminophen (Tylenol)
4. aminophylline (Truphylline)

1 3 - 8

A 17-year-old at 28 weeks gestation is having her preterm labor controlled with terbutaline (Brethine). She is to receive betamethasone valerate (Betatrex) 12 mg every 12 hours, 3 dosages. The nurse explains that the betamethasone valerate is given to:

1. reduce the client's immune response so that she does not develop pregnancy-induced hypertension (PIH).
2. enhance the baby's lung maturity by increasing the production of surfactant.
3. reduce the client's risk of infection.
4. stimulate the baby's growth so that the baby will be larger and stronger if born prematurely.

1 3 - 9

A client is scheduled to have an intravenous pyelogram (IVP). Which of the following medications must be available during this examination?

1. epinephrine (Adrenalin)
2. potassium chloride (K-Dur)
3. fludarabine (Fludara)
4. acyclovir (Zovirax)

1 3 - 1 0

Your client has been taking theophylline (Theolair-SR) but has grown weaker. The client states, "I can no longer swallow pills." Which is the best action for you to take?

1. Crush the medication and mix it with applesauce for administration.
2. Allow the client to chew the medication and "chase" it with juice.
3. Withhold the medication.
4. Consult the physician concerning a liquid form and dosage of the medication.

1 3 - 1 1

During resuscitation, your intubated client's intravenous fluid infiltrates. You know that you may deliver the following drugs via the endotracheal tube:

1. lidocaine, adenosine, naloxone, epinephrine
2. lidocaine, atropine, naloxone, norepinephrine
3. lidocaine, atropine, naloxone, epinephrine
4. lidocaine, atropine, Norcuron, epinephrine

1 3 - 1 2

Your client is a diabetic and is experiencing an attack of asthma. The physician prescribes epinephrine (Primatene). What will you teach the client about this medication?

1. Less insulin will be required, or oral hypoglycemic agents may be needed.
2. Blood pressure may be elevated, leading to danger of stroke.
3. Pupil constriction may occur, leading to decreased vision.
4. Bradycardia commonly occurs with the medication.

1 3 - 1 3

A 40-year-old client has active tuberculosis and is being treated with isoniazid (INH), streptomycin, and vitamin B_6 (pyridoxine). The client asks the nurse why pyridoxine was prescribed. The nurse explains that pyridoxine:

1. potentiates the therapeutic benefits of isoniazid.
2. reduces the risk of ototoxicity from the streptomycin.
3. reduces the peripheral neuritis associated with isoniazid.
4. prevents the recurrence of red or orange urine associated with isoniazid and streptomycin.

1 3 - 1 4

Your client has emphysema and is receiving theophylline to treat bronchospasm. You will monitor the client's serum theophylline concentration to see that the levels remain within the normal range of:

1. 10 to 20 mcg/ml.
2. 20 to 30 mcg/ml.
3. 30 to 40 mcg/ml.
4. 40 to 50 mcg/ml.

1 3 - 1 5

An older client with chronic obstructive pulmonary disease has developed pneumonia. It was determined that the causative organism is Haemophilus influenzae. You learn that the client is penicillin-allergic. You anticipate the administration of:

1. amoxicillin (Augmentin).
2. ampicillin (Omnipen).
3. trimethoprim (Trimpex).
4. ticarcillin disodium (Timentin).

1 3 - 1 6

Your 8-year-old client has cystic fibrosis and is scheduled for postural drainage. To loosen secretions and thin airway mucus, you will administer aerosol therapy containing the medication:

1. promethazine hydrochloride.
2. azithromycin.
3. Pancreatin.
4. dornase alfa.

1 3 - 1 7

Your client has a history of asthma associated with environmental allergens. To help prevent the release of the chemical mediators that cause bronchoconstriction, you anticipate the administration of:

1. cromolyn sodium.
2. theophylline.
3. aminophylline.
4. epinephrine.

1 3 - 1 8

Your client is receiving an intravenous infusion of an anti-infective to treat pneumonia. The infusion is delivering 50 ml/hour of the drug. The drop factor on the infusion set is 10 gtts/ml. You will regulate the flow at:

1. 8 gtts/min.
2. 10 gtts/min.
3. 12 gtts/min.
4. 14 gtts/min.

1 3 - 1 9

Your client has chronic obstructive pulmonary disease. To minimize the potential for contracting respiratory conditions, you will recommend that the client:

1. schedule frequent chest X rays.
2. seek immunization against influenza.
3. use diaphragmatic breathing and coughing techniques.
4. perform regular postural drainage with percussion.

1 3 - 2 0

A client with acquired immunodeficiency syndrome (AIDS) has contracted pneumocystis carinii pneumonia (PCP). You anticipate the administration of:

1. co-trimoxazole.
2. zidovudine (AZT).
3. pentamidine isethionate.
4. zalcitabine.

1 3 - 2 1

Your client has a history of motion sickness but has scheduled a cruise. To prevent the symptoms of motion sickness, the drug promethazine hydrochloride (Phenergan) has been prescribed. You will teach the client that:

1. the drug should be taken before each meal.
2. alcohol should be consumed in moderation while taking this drug.
3. the drug should not interfere with swimming and sunbathing.
4. the first dose of the drug should be taken 30 to 60 minutes before traveling.

1 3 - 2 2

A client is experiencing Legionnaires' disease. Which of the following medications would be indicated?

1. adrenalin, to relieve dyspnea
2. erythromycin, to keep the bacteria from reproducing
3. rifampin, a bacteriostatic and bactericidal agent
4. aminophylline, to relieve dyspnea due to bronchoconstriction

13-23

A client experiencing seasonal allergy symptoms is receiving triprolidine hydrochloride (Actifed). To identify the offending allergens, the client is scheduled for diagnostic skin tests (intradermal testing). You will teach the client that triprolidine hydrochloride (Actifed) should be withheld for:

1. 24 hours before the tests.
2. 48 hours before the tests.
3. 4 days before the tests.
4. 1 week before the tests.

13-24

A client recovering from a cholecystectomy received morphine sulfate in the postanesthesia care unit. When the client was returned to the surgical unit, the vital signs were: Blood pressure 124/64, pulse 64 beats per minute, respiration 8 per minute, temperature 97.4° F. Which of the following medications will the nurse anticipate administering?

1. atropine sulfate 1.0 mg IV
2. flumazenil (Romazicon) 0.2 mg IV
3. meperidine (Demerol) 50 mg IV
4. naloxone (Narcan) 0.2 mg IV

13-25

A client with chronic obstructive pulmonary disease (COPD) is receiving 1 gm of aminophylline in 1000 cc of 5% dextrose in water at 20 cc/h. Laboratory results indicate a serum aminophylline level of 25 mcg/ml. You will:

1. notify the physician.
2. increase the rate of infusion to 24 cc/h.
3. put 1 gm of aminophylline in 500 cc of D5W.
4. continue the infusion.

1 3 - 2 6

Your client was placed on aminophylline (Truphylline) 1 mg/kg/h IV for 12 hours; then 0.8 mg/kg/h to provide symptomatic relief of bronchospasm. The client is a smoker and tells you, "I think I will stop smoking." In the event the client did stop smoking, you would:

1. continue administering the medication as prescribed.
2. notify the physician that the client has stopped smoking.
3. document the fact that the client has stopped smoking.
4. decrease the amount of medication the client is taking.

1 3 - 2 7

A client is to receive cefazolin (Kefzol) to treat pneumonia. Before giving the first dose of this drug, the nurse will determine if:

1. the client is allergic to penicillin.
2. the client is allergic to yogurt or buttermilk.
3. peak and trough levels have been scheduled.
4. a chest X ray has been taken.

1 3 - 2 8

You understand that a client with a history of pulmonary impairment is not likely to be given bleomycin sulfate (Blenoxane) because this drug may cause:

1. pulmonary fibrosis.
2. an increase in vital capacity.
3. pulmonary acidosis.
4. pneumothorax.

Practice Test 13

Answers, Rationales, and Explanations

1 3 - 1

④ **Clients using the Primatene Mist inhaler should be assessed for tachycardia. Epinephrine (Primatene Mist) is an alpha and beta receptor stimulator (bronchodilator). This medication also stimulates the sympathetic nervous system and may cause tachycardia, palpitations, hypertension, and morbid (unhealthy) ventricular arrhythmias.**

1. Epinephrine (Primatene Mist) may cause hypertension, not hypotension, because it stimulates the sympathetic nervous system.
2. Epinephrine (Primatene Mist) may cause tachycardia, not bradycardia, because it stimulates the sympathetic nervous system.
3. Epinephrine (Primatene Mist) stimulates the sympathetic nervous system and may cause restlessness, nervousness, and tremors, not drowsiness.

Pregnancy Category: C

Client Need: Physiological Integrity

1 3 - 2

④ **Following the use of the beclomethasone (Beclovent) inhaler, the mouth should be rinsed well. Beclomethasone is a steroid that may cause fungal infections in the mouth due to its effect on the oral mucosa.**

1. Beclomethasone is an anti-inflammatory agent, not a bronchodilator. It is used to manage chronic conditions such as asthma. It is not indicated for use during status asthmaticus (persistent and intractable asthma).
2. Beclomethasone should be used when warmed to body temperature.
3. Beclomethasone should be taken on a regular basis, not as needed.

Pregnancy Category: C

Client Need: Health Promotion/Maintenance

1 3 - 3

④ **Terbutaline (Brethine) is a bronchodilator that acts on beta-adrenergic receptors. Because of this, the medication produces side effects of nervousness, palpitations, tremors, and tachycardia.**

1. Metoprolol (Lopressor) is a beta-blocker and therefore tends to cause drowsiness and bradycardia.
2. Alprazolam (Xanax) is an antianxiety agent and is not associated with the side effects of palpitations and insomnia.
3. Aspirin (acetylsalicylic acid) is not associated with the side effects of nervousness, palpitations, tremors, and tachycardia.

Pregnancy Category: B

Client Need: Physiological Integrity

1 3 - 4

① **Albuterol (Ventolin) may be used, along with other drugs, to treat pneumococcal pneumonia. Albuterol is a bronchodilator and exerts its bronchodilatory effect by relaxing the bronchial muscles. This relaxation is due to the drug's effect on beta receptors.**

2. Beclomethasone (Vanceril) is a steroid inhalant. This drug is used to treat the symptoms of asthma. It should not be used for clients who have bacterial infections such as pneumococcal pneumonia.

3. Ampicillin (Omnipen) is a penicillin antibiotic. It is not a bronchodilator. It is more likely that penicillin G or penicillin V would be used to treat pneumonia.

4. Acetaminophen (Tylenol) is an analgesic antipyretic, not a bronchodilator.

Pregnancy Category: C

Client Need: Physiological Integrity

1 3 - 5

② **Aminophylline (Palaron) dilates the bronchi and also increases the heart rate. Tachycardia is a frequent side effect of aminophylline.**

1. Digitalis preparations strengthen the heart rate. Aminophylline does not.

3. Nitrates dilate the coronary arteries. Aminophylline does not.

4. Calcium channel blockers will decrease myocardial oxygen demand. Aminophylline will not.

Pregnancy Category: C

Client Need: Physiological Integrity

1 3 - 6

④ **Oxygen via emergency tracheostomy at 100% is appropriate when treating airway obstruction. Some anaphylactic allergies may cause the tongue to swell. If airway obstruction occurs, the airway must be opened below the site of obstruction and oxygen delivered.**

1, 2, and 3. Oxygen via nasal cannula, facemask, and bag-valve would not be helpful because the oxygen could not get past the obstructed airway.

Pregnancy Category: NR

Client Need: Physiological Integrity

1 3 - 7

① **Intubation and 100% oxygen is appropriate when a client is apneic due to anaphylactic shock (a generalized allergic hypersensitivity of the body to a foreign protein or drug). A client experiencing anaphylaxis and respiratory arrest (apnea) requires artificial positive pressure ventilation via an endotracheal tube with 100% oxygen.**

2. Diphenhydramine (Benadryl) is an antihistamine that is useful in managing allergic reactions including anaphylaxis. However, because the client is apneic, the first consideration is to administer oxygen.

3. Acetaminophen (Tylenol) is an antipyretic and analgesic, and is not given to manage anaphylaxis or its consequence.

4. Aminophylline (Truphylline) is a bronchodilator that may be administered to manage airway obstruction due to asthma or chronic obstructive pulmonary disease. However, the priority at this time is the administration of oxygen.

Pregnancy Category: NR
Client Need: Physiological Integrity

1 3 - 8

② **Betamethasone valerate (Betatrex) is given to produce surfactant. Glucocorticoids such as betamethasone or dexamethasone administered parenterally enhance fetal lung maturity by stimulating the type II pneumocytes in the lungs to produce surfactant. The current recommendation is that betamethasone valerate 12 mg be administered to the mother every 12 hours for a minimum of 3 dosages, or dexamethasone 5 mg every 12 hours for a maximum of 4 doses.**

1. Betamethasone valerate (Betatrex) is a glucocorticoid and has no impact on pregnancy-induced hypertension.

3. Betamethasone valerate (Betatrex) is a glucocorticoid and has no impact on the immune system to reduce risk of infection.

4. Betamethasone valerate (Betatrex) enhances lung maturity, not the growth of the fetus.

Pregnancy Category: C
Client Need: Health Promotion/Maintenance

1 3 - 9

① **Epinephrine (Adrenalin) must be available for clients having an intravenous pyelogram (IVP). Epinephrine (Adrenalin) is a bronchodilator and cardiac stimulant administered to manage anaphylaxis due to hypersensitivity to the contrast medium used for intravenous pyelogram (IVP). An intravenous pyelogram is a diagnostic test used to visualize the renal system and assess its function. A radiopaque dye is injected into the veins of the client. Because anaphylaxis has occasionally occurred in response to the dye, resuscitation equipment and drugs such as epinephrine must be available.**

2. Potassium chloride (K-Dur) is administered to manage potassium depletion. This client does not demonstrate a need for this medication.

3. Fludarabine (Fludara) is administered to manage Hodgkin's lymphoma and chronic lymphocytic leukemia. This client does not have either of these conditions.

4. Acyclovir (Zovirax) is an antiviral agent. This client does not demonstrate a need for this type of medication.

Pregnancy Category: C
Client Need: Health Promotion/Maintenance

13-10

④ **A liquid should be given. Theophylline (Theolair-SR) comes in liquid form and the dosage can be adjusted if clients are unable to swallow the tablet/capsule. Theolair-SR (sustained release) is a bronchodilator used in the treatment of airway obstruction associated with asthma or obstructive pulmonary disease.**

1 and 2. Sustained-release medications should not be crushed or chewed. If sustained-release medications are crushed or chewed, the sustaining mechanism of the medication will be compromised.

3. The client needs the medication. It is the route of administration that should be changed.

Pregnancy Category: C

Client Need: Physiological Integrity

13-11

③ **Lidocaine, atropine, naloxone, and epinephrine are medications used for resuscitation. They may all be given via the endotracheal tube should it become necessary.**

1, 2, and 4. Adenosine, norepinephrine, and Norcuron may only be given intravenously.

Pregnancy Category: lidocaine, B; atropine, C; naloxone, B; epinephrine, C

Client Need: Safe, Effective Care Environment

13-12

② **You would teach the client about elevated blood pressure and the danger of stroke. Clients receiving epinephrine (Primatene) should be taught to assess their blood pressure. Epinephrine (Primatene) is a sympathomimetic drug. Because of its impact on the sympathetic nervous system, vasoconstriction, tachycardia, and hypertension may occur.**

1. Taking epinephrine (Primatene) may lead to a need for increased dosages of insulin/oral hypoglycemics in clients with diabetes.

3. Sympathomimetics such as epinephrine dilate pupils.

4. Sympathomimetics such as epinephrine tend to cause tachyarrhythmias, not bradycardia.

Pregnancy Category: C

Client Need: Health Promotion/Maintenance

1 3 - 1 3

③ Vitamin B₆ (pyridoxine) reduces the side effects of isoniazid therapy. A side effect of isoniazid therapy is peripheral neuritis (inflammation of a nerve or nerves). The coadministration of pyridoxine (B₆, a water-soluble vitamin) reduces the unpleasantness of this side effect for the client.

1. Pyridoxine does not potentiate or cause a synergistic action between isoniazid and streptomycin.

2. Risks associated with the use of streptomycin are ototoxicity, hepatotoxicity, and nephrotoxicity. Vitamin B₆ does not protect against ototoxicity, since hearing damage is associated with cranial nerve damage rather than peripheral nerve damage.

4. Red or orange urine is a side effect associated with rifampin, not streptomycin and isoniazid. Rifampin may also be prescribed for the treatment of tuberculosis. Rifampin not only changes the urine to a reddish-orange when administered over a period of time, but the color of perspiration, tears, saliva, and feces are also affected.

Pregnancy Category: A
Client Need: Psychosocial Integrity

1 3 - 1 4

① Serum theophylline levels should range between 10 and 20 mcg/ml. Levels above 20 mcg/ml are associated with signs of toxicity that include: Tachycardia, anorexia, nausea, vomiting, diarrhea, restlessness, and headache. Theophylline is a bronchodilator used to treat acute and chronic bronchospasms.

2, 3, and 4. Serum theophylline levels above 20 mcg/ml will produce signs of toxicity.

Pregnancy Category: C
Client Need: Physiological Integrity

1 3 - 1 5

③ You will anticipate administering the anti-infective trimethoprim (Trimpex). Trimethoprim would be an appropriate choice for clients who are penicillin-allergic and have bacterial pneumonia caused by Haemophilus influenzae.

1. Amoxicillin (Augmentin) is a penicillin and would not be administered due to this client's allergy to penicillin.

2. Ampicillin (Omnipen) is a penicillin and would not be administered due to this client's allergy to penicillin.

4. Ticarcillin disodium (Timentin) is a penicillin and would not be given due to the client's allergy to penicillin.

Pregnancy Category: C
Client Need: Health Promotion/Maintenance

1 3 - 1 6

④ **You will administer dornase alfa (Pulmozyme). This medication is a genetically engineered pulmonary enzyme. It is administered prior to postural drainage by an aerosol nebulizer and effectively loosens secretions and thins airway mucus.**

1. Promethazine hydrochloride is an antihistamine and would be contraindicated due to its drying effect on mucous membranes. Expectoration is hindered when membranes are dry. Also, this medication is not available as an aerosol.

2. Azithromycin is a broad-spectrum anti-infective. It could be prescribed to help control infection. However, it does not loosen secretions or thin airway mucus.

3. Pancreatin is a digestive enzyme that would be administered to treat the deficiency of pancreatic enzymes such as those associated with cystic fibrosis. However, it does not loosen secretions or thin airway mucus.

Pregnancy Category: B

Client Need: Physiological Integrity

1 3 - 1 7

① **You would anticipate the administration of cromolyn sodium (Nasalcrom). Cromolyn sodium helps to prevent the release of chemical mediators such as histamine and leukotrienes that would otherwise cause bronchodilation. It is prescribed to help prevent mild to moderate asthma associated with environmental allergens.**

2. Theophylline is a bronchodilator that is given to treat bronchospasm. It is not administered to prevent bronchoconstriction caused by environmental allergens.

3. Aminophylline is a bronchodilator that is given for the symptomatic relief of bronchospasm. It is not administered to prevent bronchospasm, nor is it administered to prevent bronchoconstriction caused by environmental allergens.

4. Epinephrine is a bronchodilator and is associated with the treatment of acute asthma and status asthmaticus.

Pregnancy Category: B

Client Need: Health Promotion/Maintenance

1 3 - 1 8

① **To determine the correct drip rate, multiply the hourly amount (50) times the drop factor (10). Divide the answer (500) by 60 minutes.**

$$\frac{50 \times 10}{60 \text{ min}} = \frac{500}{60} = 8 \text{ gtts / min}$$

2. 10 gtts/min would be too fast.

3. 12 gtts/min would be too fast.

4. 14 gtts/min would be too fast.

Pregnancy Category: NA

Client Need: Physiological Integrity

13-19

② **You will encourage the client to seek immunization against influenza and streptococcus pneumoniae. Clients with chronic obstructive pulmonary disease are prone to respiratory conditions.**

1. Scheduling frequent X rays will not minimize the client's potential for contracting respiratory conditions. Chest X rays are diagnostic (they do not prevent or treat conditions).

3. Diaphragmatic breathing and coughing techniques help to improve ventilation and produce secretions without causing breathlessness and fatigue. However, these techniques do not directly lower the client's potential for contracting certain respiratory conditions, as would an immunization program.

4. Performing regular postural drainage with percussion will help raise secretions. However, postural drainage will not directly lower the client's potential for contracting certain respiratory conditions. An immunization program directly helps prevent specific respiratory conditions.

Pregnancy Category: C
Client Need: Health Promotion/Maintenance

13-20

③ **You will anticipate administering the drug pentamidine isethionate. This drug is an anti-infective/amebicide/antiprotozoal. The organism responsible for pneumocystis carinii pneumonia is the P. carinii protozoon. It is normally present in the lungs of humans and various animals. However, it becomes an aggressive pathogen in the immunocompromised client.**

1. Co-trimoxazole is among the drugs of choice for treating pneumocystis carinii. However, pentamidine isethionate may produce less severe adverse reactions in clients who are immunocompromised.

2. Zidovudine (AZT) is administered to treat acquired immunodeficiency syndrome, not pneumocystis carinii pneumonia. Also, zidovudine is an antiviral, not an anti-infective.

4. Zalcitabine (HIVID) is an antiviral drug administered to treat clients with advanced HIV disease who cannot tolerate the drug zidovudine. It has no effect on pneumocystis carinii pneumonia.

Pregnancy Category: C
Client Need: Physiological Integrity

1 3 - 2 1

④ **You will teach the client to take the first dose of the antihistamine promethazine hydrochloride (Phenergan) 30 to 60 minutes prior to travel. The object is to prevent the symptoms of motion sickness. Once the symptoms have begun, they are more difficult to treat.**

1. When promethazine hydrochloride (Phenergan) is administered to prevent/treat the symptoms of motion sickness, it should be taken upon arising and again with the evening meal.

2. Alcohol should be avoided until the client knows the extent of the drug's effect on the central nervous system. The client should also be warned to avoid activities that require alertness while taking the drug.

3. Clients taking promethazine hydrochloride (Phenergan) should be taught that photosensitivity and rash may occur. A sunscreen lotion should be applied and the client should wear protective clothing.

Pregnancy Category: C
Client Need: Health Promotion/Maintenance

1 3 - 2 2

② **Erythromycin is the drug of choice for the treatment of Legionnaires' disease because it is bacteriostatic (keeps the bacteria Legionella pneumophila from reproducing). Legionnaires' disease is a severe and sometimes fatal disease characterized by pneumonia, dry cough, myalgia, and occasionally gastrointestinal (GI) symptoms.**

1. Adrenalin relieves dyspnea due to bronchoconstriction by relaxing the smooth muscles of the bronchial tree. However, it has no direct impact on Legionnaires' disease.

3. Rifampin may be added to the treatment of Legionnaires' disease in severe cases, but it should never be given to resistant organisms developing during monotherapy. It is bacteriostatic and bactericidal and is also given to treat tuberculosis.

4. Aminophylline is a bronchodilator. It relieves dyspnea due to bronchoconstriction, but, like adrenalin, will not keep organisms from reproducing.

Pregnancy Category: B
Client Need: Physiological Integrity

1 3 - 2 3

③ **You will teach the client that the triprolidine hydrochloride (Actifed) should be withheld starting 4 days before skin tests (intradermal testing) are scheduled. Antihistamines such as Actifed can prevent, reduce, or mask positive skin test results.**

1 and 2. Waiting as late as 24 to 48 hours before the skin tests to discontinue the Actifed would most likely invalidate the skin test results.

4. It would not be necessary to discontinue the Actifed as much as 1 week before the skin tests.

Pregnancy Category: C
Client Need: Physiological Integrity

13-24

④ **The nurse will anticipate a prescription for naloxone (Narcan). Naloxone (Narcan) is a narcotic agonist administered to treat oversedation from narcotic analgesics. A respiratory rate < 12/min is a sign of respiratory depression, most likely due to the morphine sulfate administered in the postanesthesia area.**

1. Atropine sulfate may be prescribed to treat bradycardia (heart rate < 60). It is not prescribed to treat respiratory depression.

2. Flumazenil (Romazicon) is a benzodiazepine antagonist and may be prescribed to treat overdoses of medications like diazepam (Valium).

3. Meperidine (Demerol) should not be given. It is a narcotic analgesic and would further depress respirations.

Pregnancy Category: B
Client Need: Physiological Integrity

13-25

① **The physician should be notified because the client's serum aminophylline level is abnormally high. The therapeutic range for aminophylline is 10 to 20 mcg/ml.**

2 and 3. Infusing more of the aminophylline by increasing the drops per minute or the concentration will elevate the serum aminophylline level further.

4. The infusion should be stopped and the physician notified.

Pregnancy Category: C
Client Need: Health Promotion/Maintenance

13-26

② **You would notify the physician that the client has stopped smoking. Smoking constricts blood vessels. Clients who smoke and are taking the bronchodilator aminophylline (Truphylline) will require more of the drug to bring about the relief of bronchospasm. Nonsmokers will require less of the drug.**

1. The nurse should withhold the aminophylline (Truphylline) and notify the physician that the client has stopped smoking. Nonsmokers require less of the medication than do smokers.

3. Simply documenting the fact that the client has stopped smoking will not protect the client from the unnecessarily large amount of the drug administered. The dosage should be decreased.

4. The nurse should anticipate that the drug dosage will be decreased. However, the nurse would not decrease the dosage without notifying the physician that this client has stopped smoking.

Pregnancy Category: C
Client Need: Physiological Integrity

1 3 - 2 7

1. ① Before administering the first dosage of cefazolin (Kefzol), the client should be assessed for an allergy to penicillin. Cefazolin (Kefzol) is a first-generation cephalosporin. There can be a cross-allergy between penicillins and cephalosporins.

2. Allergies to yogurt or buttermilk would not prevent the administration of cefazolin.

3. Peak and trough levels are appropriate with aminoglycosides, not first-generation cephalosporins such as Kefzol.

4. Blood and other cultures should be completed before beginning antibiotics, but not necessarily a chest X ray.

Pregnancy Category: B
Client Need: Health Promotion/Maintenance

1 3 - 2 8

1. ① Clients with a history of pulmonary impairment should not receive bleomycin sulfate (Blenoxane) since pulmonary fibrosis may occur.

2. There may be a decrease, not increase, in vital capacity due to the possibility of pulmonary fibrosis.

3. Pulmonary alkalosis, not acidosis, is likely to occur since carbon dioxide may build up.

4. Pneumothorax (a collection of air or gas in the pleural cavity) is associated with a perforation through the chest wall.

Pregnancy Category: D
Client Need: Health Promotion/Maintenance

Practice Test 14

Topical Agents

OVERVIEW

Topical agents treat and inhibit conditions associated with a defined area of the body, such as the skin and hair.

Topical agents include:

- **Local anesthetics**
- **Local anti-infectives**
- **Scabicides and pediculicides**
- **Topical corticosteroids**

LOCAL ANESTHETICS

Local anesthetics create partial or complete loss of sensation without loss of consciousness. Local anesthetics produce brief effects by slowing down nerve transmission only in the areas where they are applied or injected.

Local anesthetics include:

- Benzocaine (Americaine)
- Lidocaine (Prilocaine)

Conditions treated with local anesthetics include:

- Hemorrhoidal discomfort
- Stitch cuts
- Warts, in surgical removal

LOCAL ANTI-INFECTIVES

Local anti-infectives are administered to treat various infections limited to one place or area on the body. They are normally available as ointments, creams, lotions, gels, pledgets, solutions, shampoos, powders, and sprays.

Local anti-infectives include:

- Butoconazole nitrate (Femstat)
- Gentamicin sulfate (Garamycin)

Conditions treated with local anti-infectives include:

- Superficial burns, abrasions
- Vulvovaginal infections caused by Candida

SCABICIDES AND PEDICULICIDES

SCABICIDES kill mites, especially those associated with scabies (a highly communicable skin disease caused by an arachnid).

Scabicides include:

Lindane (Kwell)

PEDICULICIDES are substances that kill lice.

Pediculicides include:

- Permethrin (Nix)

Conditions treated with scabicides and pediculicides include:

- Parasite infestation (scabies)
- Pediculosis capitis (head lice)
- Pediculosis corporis (body lice)

TOPICAL CORTICOSTEROIDS

Topical corticosteroids interfere with the inflammation and pruritus associated with various conditions. Topical corticosteroids exhibit anti-inflammatory, antipruritic, vasoconstrictive, and antiproliferative activity.

Topical corticosteroids include:

- Hydrocortisone (Cortizone)
- Hydrocortisone acetate (Cortaid)

Conditions treated with topical corticosteroids include:

- Inflammation and pruritus associated with corticosteroid-responsive dermatoses
- Seborrheic dermatitis of the scalp

Practice Test 14

Questions

1 4 - 1

The parents of a 3-year-old notice head lice on their child. Lindane (Kwell) shampoo is to be used for treatment. The nurse instructs the parents that Kwell should be used carefully with small children due to an increased risk for:

1. ototoxicity.
2. neurotoxicity.
3. nephrotoxicity.
4. hepatoxicity.

1 4 - 2

Your client has a partial-thickness burn. Which of the following topical medications would be appropriate?

1. silver sulfadiazine (Silvadene)
2. ketoconazole (Nizoral)
3. metronidazole (MetroGel)
4. nitroglycerin (glyceryl trinitrate)

1 4 - 3

Parents of pediatric clients who have chicken-pox should be advised to avoid administering:

1. calamine lotion over or around lesions.
2. acetaminophen (Tylenol) by mouth for fever and pain.
3. diphenhydramine (Benadryl) by mouth for itch.
4. diphenhydramine (Benadryl) ointment liberally over the whole body.

1 4 - 4

Your client is receiving initial therapy to treat herpes genitalis. Acyclovir ointment 5% will be administered. You will teach the client that:

1. virus transmission can occur during treatment.
2. the ointment will heal the lesions.
3. it is not necessary to cover the entire lesion with the ointment.
4. the acyclovir treatment can begin at any time while the condition is active.

1 4 - 5

A 7-year-old received third-degree burns to both hands following an accident involving firecrackers. Mafenide acetate (Sulfamylon) cream will be applied bid. You know the purpose of this drug is to:

1. stimulate growth of tissue.
2. prevent loss of tissue fluid.
3. inhibit the growth of pathogenic organisms.
4. depress transmission of pain impulses.

1 4 - 6

An older adult is experiencing acne vulgaris. Which of the following medications would you administer to treat this condition?

1. bacitracin ointment (Baciguent).
2. azelaic acid cream (Azelex).
3. Fungizone cream (amphotericin B).
4. acyclovir ointment (Zovirax).

1 4 - 7

A male client comes to the clinic and tells the nurse, "I need to get some medicine for jock itch." The nurse will anticipate a prescription for the medication:

1. bacitracin (Baciguent)
2. gentamicin sulfate (G-myticin)
3. amphotericin B (Fungizone)
4. metronidazole (MetroCream)

1 4 - 8

Your client is experiencing vulvovaginal candidiasis and is to receive the medication tioconazole (Vagistat-1). Which comment by the client indicates she understands how to administer this medication?

1. "I will open the application 10 to 15 minutes before I use it, to allow it to get warm."
2. "It is OK for me to have sex after I have inserted the medication."
3. "It is not necessary for me to use the medication during my menstrual period."
4. "I should insert the medication high in my vagina."

1 4 - 9

A male client comes to the clinic complaining of itching under his beard. It has been determined that he has tinea barbae. To treat this condition, the drug sulconazole nitrate (Exelderm) will be administered. You will inform the client that his symptoms should be relieved within:

1. 12 to 24 hours.
2. a few days.
3. 1 to 2 weeks.
4. 2 to 4 weeks.

1 4 - 1 0

A toddler has impetigo contagiosa (staphylococcus) and will receive mupirocin (Bactroban) applications tid for 1 to 2 weeks. You will teach the parents to notify the physician if no improvement occurs within:

1. 1 to 2 days.
2. 3 to 5 days.
3. 7 to 10 days.
4. 14 to 21 days.

Practice Test 14

Answers, Rationales, and Explanations

1 4 - 1

② Kwell shampoo should be used carefully in children since it penetrates the skin and can damage nerve tissue (be neurotoxic). The younger the child, the more permeable the skin. Kwell should be administered cautiously in children under the age of 10, but particularly in infants, small children, and those with preexisting seizure disorders. Children with seizure disorders have an increased risk for neurotoxicity.

1, 3, and 4. Lindane (Kwell) is not ototoxic (damaging to the auditory nerve—8th cranial nerve), nephrotoxic (damaging to kidney tissue), or hepatotoxic (damaging to liver tissue).

Pregnancy Category: B
Client Need: Safe, Effective Care Environment

1 4 - 2

① You will anticipate a prescription for silver sulfadiazine (Silvadene). Silvadene is a broad-spectrum antibiotic cream used to prevent or treat wound infections in partial-thickness burns.

2. Ketoconazole (Nizoral) is an antifungal cream/shampoo whose uses include the treatment of seborrheic dermatitis (dandruff).
3. Metronidazole (MetroGel) is a topical or vaginal gel used to treat bacterial vaginosis.
4. Nitroglycerin (glyceryl trinitrate 2%) is a topical nitroglycerin ointment used to treat angina.

Pregnancy Category: B
Client Need: Physiological Integrity

1 4 - 3

④ The parents of children who have chickenpox should not put diphenhydramine (Benadryl) liberally over their children's bodies. Diphenhydramine (Benadryl) is an antihistamine that is very useful in relieving local skin irritation when applied topically, due to its impact on the inflammatory response. It is, however, absorbed systemically, especially if open lesions are present. Dosage may be excessive if the ointment is applied too liberally.

1. Calamine lotion is a drying agent and may help to dry up the lesions and promote healing.
2. Acetaminophen (Tylenol) is an analgesic antipyretic that will provide comfort during the acute phase of the illness.
3. Diphenhydramine (Benadryl) by mouth may provide relief from the discomfort of chickenpox.

Pregnancy Category: B
Client Need: Physiological Integrity

1 4 - 4

(1) **You will teach the client that viral transmission of herpes genitalis can occur during treatment. The acyclovir ointment should be applied with a finger cot or rubber glove to prevent autoinoculation (spread of the herpes virus from one part of a client's body to another part of the client's body). Health-care providers can also be infected by this highly contagious disease and should use appropriate universal precautions.**

2. Acyclovir is not a cure for herpes genitalis, but it does treat the symptoms, which include: Itching, soreness, and pain.

3. The acyclovir ointment should be applied over the entire area of the lesions and all lesions should be covered thoroughly.

4. Therapy with acyclovir ointment should begin as soon as the signs and symptoms of the condition appear.

Pregnancy Category: C

Client Need: Physiological Integrity

1 4 - 5

(3) **You know that the purpose of mafenide acetate (Sulfamylon) is to inhibit the growth of pathogenic organisms. It is a topical anti-infective that kills bacteria by interfering with their cellular metabolism.**

1. Mafenide acetate (Sulfamylon) is a local anti-infective. It facilitates tissue growth indirectly by promoting an environment free of infection.

2. Tissue fluid loss is not affected by mafenide acetate (Sulfamylon).

4. To treat pain, an analgesic would be required, not an anti-infective.

Pregnancy Category: C

Client Need: Physiological Integrity

1 4 - 6

(2) **You would administer the local anti-infective azelaic acid cream (Azelex) for the treatment of acne vulgaris. The action of this drug is unknown; however, it may inhibit microbial cellular protein synthesis. The cream should be thoroughly massaged into the affected area bid. The face, neck, and shoulders are common sites. Acne vulgaris is a common acne, presenting papules, pustules, or hypertrophied nodules caused by overgrowth of connective tissue.**

1. Bacitracin (Baciguent) is a bactericidal or bacteriostatic, depending on the organism being treated and the concentration of the drug. It inhibits bacterial cell-wall synthesis. It is used for topical infections, abrasions, cuts, and minor burns or wounds.

3. Fungizone cream (amphotericin B) is indicated for cutaneous or mucocutaneous candidal infections. Candida is a yeastlike fungus.

4. Acyclovir (Zovirax) ointment is indicated for initial herpes genitalis. Apply with finger cot or rubber gloves. Acyclovir is not a cure but will help ease the symptoms.

Pregnancy Category: B

Client Need: Health Promotion/Maintenance

1 4 - 7

③   **The nurse will anticipate a prescription for amphotericin B (Fungizone). This medica-tion is a local anti-infective (an agent that kills fungi and spores) and is commonly administered to treat skin diseases such as the infection candidiasis (jock itch). Fungizone is available as a cream, lotion, and ointment.**

1.   Bacitracin (Baciguent) is a bacteriostatic or bactericidal that is administered to treat topical infections, abrasions, cuts, and minor burns or wounds. It is available as an ointment (500 units/gm).

2.   Gentamicin sulfate (G-myticin) is a local anti-infective administered to treat bacterial infec-tions, such as superficial burns of the skin. It is available as a cream or ointment.

4.   Metronidazole (MetroCream) is an anti-infective administered to treat the inflammatory papules and pustules associated with acne rosacea.

Pregnancy Category: B

Client Need: Physiological Integrity

1 4 - 8

④   **The client understands how to administer tioconazole (Vagistat-1) if she indicates that she should insert it high in the vagina. Inserting the medication high in the vagina will allow it to come in contact with the infected areas of the vagina.**

1.   The application of tioconazole (Vagistat-1) should be opened just before use in order to prevent contamination of the ointment.

2.   A client with vulvovaginal candidiasis should be taught to avoid sexual intercourse on the night she inserts the Vagistat-1 and the night after insertion, unless her partner uses a condom to prevent reinfection.

3.   A full course of tioconazole (Vagistat-1) should be completed, including during the client's menstrual period.

Pregnancy Category: C

Client Need: Physiological Integrity

1 4 - 9

②   **The client will be taught that clinical improvement is normally noticed within 1 week and symptomatic relief within a few days.**

1.   It takes longer than 12 to 24 hours for clients to experience symptomatic relief from tinea barbae.

3 and 4. Symptomatic relief from tinea barbae should be manifested before 1 to 4 weeks after the topical application of sulconazole nitrate (Exelderm). If no improvement occurs after 4 weeks, diagnosis should be reconsidered.

Pregnancy Category: C

Client Need: Physiological Integrity

1 4 - 1 0

② **Parents should be taught to notify the physician if there is no improvement within 3 to 5 days. Applications of a 2% ointment of mupirocin (Bactroban) should bring improvement within 3 to 5 days to clients who have impetigo. This drug is thought to inhibit bacterial (staphylococcus) protein and RNA synthesis.**

1. It is unlikely that noticeable improvement will occur within 12 to 24 hours of the administration of mupirocin (Bactroban).

3 and 4. Parents should not wait 7 to 21 days after the application of mupirocin (Bactroban) to notify the physician that no improvement has occurred.

Pregnancy Category: B

Client Need: Physiological Integrity

Practice Test 15

Miscellaneous Medications

OVERVIEW

The "miscellaneous" category comprises drugs that are of mixed character. Among the miscellaneous drugs are agents that are uncategorized.

Miscellaneous agents include:

- Antigout substances
- Diagnostic skin tests
- Enzymes
- Gold salts
- Miscellaneous antagonists and antidotes
- Spasmolytics
- Uterine substances

ANTIGOUT SUBSTANCES

Antigout substances are administered to treat the symptoms of gout, which are caused by the deposit of urate crystals in the joints. Antigout substances function in three general ways: They reduce the production of uric acid, reduce inflammation, and increase the excretion of uric acid by the kidneys.

Antigout substances include:

- Allopurinol (Zyloprim)
- Colchicine (Colgout)
- Probenecid (Benemid)

Conditions treated with antigout substances include:

- Gouty arthritis
- Hyperuricemia secondary to malignancies

DIAGNOSTIC SKIN TESTS

Diagnostic skin tests such as the tuberculin purified protein derivative (PPD Mantoux, ST) are used to determine if a client has a specific disease; i.e., tuberculosis.

Diagnostic skin tests include:

- Tuberculin purified protein derivative histoplasmin

Conditions treated with diagnostic skin tests include:

- Histoplasmosis
- Mumps
- Tuberculosis

ENZYMES

Enzymes are complex proteins capable of inducing chemical changes in other substances without being changed themselves. Enzymes act as organic catalysts in initiating or speeding up specific chemical reactions.

Enzymes include:

- Chymopapain (Chymodiactin)
- Hyaluronidase (Wydase)

Conditions treated with enzymes include:

- Inflammatory and infected lesions (in debridement)
- Herniated lumbar disk
- Enzymes are also administered as adjunct therapy to increase absorption and dispersion of injected drugs.

GOLD SALTS

Gold salts are derived from gold (chemical symbol Au).

Gold salts include:

- Auranofin (Ridaura)
- Gold sodium thiomalate (Aurolate)

Conditions treated with gold salts include:

- Rheumatoid arthritis

MISCELLANEOUS ANTAGONISTS AND ANTIDOTES

Antagonists and antidotes are usually administered to counteract the action of something or neutralize poisons or the effects of poisons.

Miscellaneous antagonists include:

- Dimercaprol (BAL in Oil)
- Edetate disodium (Disotate)

Conditions treated with antagonists include:

- Arsenic or gold poisoning
- Hypercalcemic crisis

Miscellaneous antidotes include:

- Activated charcoal
- Digoxin immune Fab (ovine) (Digibind)

Conditions treated with antidotes include:

- Life-threatening intoxication with digitoxin or digoxin
- Overdosage of acetaminophen

SPASMOLYTICS

Spasmolytics are administered to relieve muscle spasms.

Spasmolytics include:

- Flavoxate hydrochloride (Urispas)
- Oxybutynin chloride (Ditropan)

Conditions treated with spasmolytics include:

- Neurogenic bladder
- Dysuria, for symptomatic relief

UTERINE SUBSTANCES

Three types of substances are administered for their effects on the uterus:

(1) Oxytocics

(2) Uterine relaxants

(3) Abortifacients

OXYTOCIC substances stimulate the uterus.

Oxytocic agents include:

- Methylergonovine maleate (Methergine)
- Oxytocin (Pitocin)

Conditions treated with oxytocics include:

- Postpartum uterine bleeding
- Uterine atony

UTERINE RELAXANTS are administered to soothe and relax the muscles of the uterus. They are administered to prevent the potential for abortion and miscarriage.

Uterine relaxants include:

- Terbutaline sulfate (Brethine)
- Magnesium sulfate

Conditions treated with uterine relaxants include:

■ Threatened abortion

ABORTIFACIENTS are used to cause or induce an abortion.

Abortifacients include:

■ RU 486 (Mifepristone)   ■ Prostaglandin gel

Conditions treated with abortifacients include:

■ Pregnancy, to induce therapeutic abortion

■ Pregnancy, to induce elective abortion

Practice Test 15

Questions

1 5 - 1

Your client was given a Purified Protein Derivative (PPD) on the inside of the forearm 48 hours ago. A 12-mm induration has developed. You know this indicates:

1. active tuberculosis.
2. immunity to tuberculosis.
3. advanced tuberculosis.
4. exposure to tuberculosis.

1 5 - 2

Your client is receiving ritodrine hydrochloride (Yutopar) intravenously. With the initiation of this drug, it is most important to assess for any adverse reactions that could affect:

1. uterine function.
2. gastrointestinal function.
3. central nervous system function.
4. cardiac function.

1 5 - 3

A postoperative client has been medicated for pain with a long-acting narcotic. You notice that the client's respiratory rate is 8 breaths per minute. For which medication do you anticipate a prescription?

1. meperidine (Demerol)
2. promethazine (Phenergan)
3. naloxone (Narcan)
4. flumazenil (Romazicon)

1 5 - 4

Your client has heparin toxicity. You will anticipate administering which one of the following medications?

1. warfarin (Coumadin)
2. vitamin K
3. digoxin
4. protamine sulfate

1 5 - 5

A client experiencing gout may receive which of the following medications?

1. furosemide (Lasix)
2. colchicine
3. prochlorperazine (Compazine)
4. potassium chloride (K-Dur)

1 5 - 6

A client age 16 was brought to the Emergency Department unconscious as a result of heroin overdose. The nurse will anticipate administering which one of the following medications?

1. triazolam (Halcion)
2. diazepam (Valium)
3. naloxone (Narcan)
4. haloperidol (Haldol)

1 5 - 7

An agitated client has 5 mg of diazepam (Valium) prescribed intravenously every 2 hours as needed. After administering a dose, you observe that the client's respiratory rate has changed from 20/min to 6/min. You anticipate a prescription for:

1. fentanyl (Sublimaze)
2. fluorouracil (Adrucil)
3. fluconasole (Diflucan)
4. flumazenil (Romazicon)

15-8

A client experiencing urticaria might benefit most from a prescription for which one of the following medications?

1. diphenhydramine (Benadryl) 25 mg by mouth
2. sulconazole nitrate (Exelderm) cream
3. terconazole (Terazol) suppositories
4. tetracycline hydrochloride (Topicycline) ointment

15-9

A client with gout has been placed on a medication to facilitate excretion of uric acid. Which of the following medications would have the effects of promoting resorption of tissue deposits and excretion of uric acid?

1. colchicine
2. metolazone (Zaroxolyn)
3. probenecid (Benemid)
4. allopurinol (Zyloprim)

15-10

To prevent acetaldehyde syndrome, the drug disulfiram (Antabuse) should not be administered to clients who have consumed alcohol within the last:

1. 12 hours.
2. 24 hours.
3. 36 hours.
4. 48 hours.

15-11

Which of the following poisonous ingestions or overdoses should not be treated with syrup of ipecac?

1. acetaminophen
2. gentamicin
3. multivitamins
4. petroleum-based products

1 5 - 1 2

Your client is receiving a heparin infusion. The morning laboratory report reveals: PTT 246 sec, K+ 4.6 mmol/l, Na+ 136 mmol/l. You anticipate the administration of:

1. promethazine.
2. protamine sulfate.
3. procainamide.
4. propranolol.

1 5 - 1 3

A client with gout is receiving colchicine and allopurinol (Zyloprim). Which of the following symptoms will the nurse recognize as potential side effects of antigout therapy?

1. epistaxis, bruising, and petechiae
2. constipation, neuropathic leg
3. tinnitus, blurred vision
4. warmth and feelings of flushing

1 5 - 1 4

Oxytocin (Pitocin) is being given intravenously to enhance labor in a 30-year-old primigravida. The nurse's assessment reveals the following: Contractions 3 minutes apart and lasting 55 seconds, fetal heart rate at 130 dropping to 90–100 during contractions and returning to baseline, and maternal urinary output averaging 40 cc/hour. Which of the following would the nurse consider as normal in this primigravida during Pitocin administration?

1. contractions less than 2 minutes apart
2. contractions lasting 60 to 90 seconds or longer
3. painful contractions and increased uterine activity
4. drowsiness and headache

15-15

Receiving treatment with radioactive iodine would be contraindicated in which of the following?

1. pregnancy
2. hyperthyroidism
3. clients over 50 years of age
4. presence of a goiter

15-16

Which statement made by a client indicates a correct understanding of the medication lindane (Kwell) shampoo?

1. "I will need to apply this shampoo daily for 2 weeks."
2. "None of the members of my family will have to use the shampoo."
3. "This shampoo will treat my head lice as well as my dandruff condition."
4. "It is important for me to comb my hair with a fine-toothed comb since the shampoo won't remove all the nits."

15-17

Serum uric acid levels are elevated to 8 mg/dl in a client experiencing great-toe pain. Which of the following medications would you give?

1. penicillin G potassium (Pfizerpen)
2. aspirin (acetylsalicylic acid)
3. acetaminophen (Tylenol)
4. allopurinol (Zyloprim)

Practice Test 15

Answers, Rationales, and Explanations

15-1

④ **You understand that the client has been exposed to tuberculosis.** A 12-mm induration indicates that the client has been exposed to Mycobacterium tuberculosis recently or in the past. It does not necessarily suggest that the client has active tubercular disease. This reaction might be due to actual disease or exposure to the disease. Diagnosis of pulmonary tuberculosis is usually confirmed by chest X ray and sputum tests.

1. Active tuberculosis is not diagnosed by the tubercle extract injection. A significant skin-test reaction (10 mm or more) would be followed up by sputum testing and chest X ray.

2. A positive result of the tubercle bacillus extract injection does not imply immunity to tuberculosis.

3. Advanced tuberculosis is not diagnosed by the tubercle bacillus extract injection.

Pregnancy Category: C

Client Need: Health Promotion/Maintenance

15-2

④ **You should assess for adverse reactions affecting cardiac function.** When administering ritodrine hydrochloride (Yutopar), you will observe cardiac function. The administration of ritodrine hydrochloride (Yutopar) is associated with cardiovascular side effects such as tachycardia, palpitations, premature ventricular contractions, and widening pulse pressure. These effects are the most important to assess since they may be life threatening.

1. Ritodrine hydrochloride (Yutopar) is administered to inhibit uterine contractibility in the management of preterm labor; however, cardiovascular side effects are the most important to assess when the drug is first initiated.

2. Ritodrine hydrochloride (Yutopar), when administered by mouth, should be given with meals to reduce the potential for nausea and vomiting. However, assessing cardiac function is the priority.

3. Even though ritodrine hydrochloride (Yutopar) may cause anxiety and nervousness, it is the assessment of cardiovascular effects that is the most critical.

Pregnancy Category: B

Client Need: Physiological Integrity

15-3

③ **Naloxone (Narcan) is a narcotic antagonist (prevents cells from responding by binding to them) used to treat narcotic overdose with accompanying respiratory depression.**

1. Meperidine (Demerol) is a narcotic analgesic and would depress respirations further.

2. Promethazine (Phenergan) is an antiemetic that may potentiate the action of narcotics.

4. Flumazenil (Romazicon) is a benzodiazepine antagonist (that is, it counteracts the action of benzodiazepine) used to treat benzodiazepine overdose.

Pregnancy Category: B

Client Need: Health Promotion/Maintenance

1 5 - 4

④ **You will administer protamine sulfate. Protamine sulfate is a heparin antagonist (antidote) given intravenously that combines with heparin to form an inactive substance. Protamine sulfate may be given for extremely elevated partial thromboplastin time (PTT).**

1. Warfarin is an anticoagulant and would therefore be inappropriate to administer.
2. Vitamin K is the antidote for warfarin toxicity.
3. Digoxin is a cardiac glycoside.

Pregnancy Category: C
Client Need: Physiological Integrity

1 5 - 5

② **Colchicine is an antigout medication that reduces uric acid production, thus reducing the deposit of uric acid crystals in the joints. Gout is a hereditary metabolic disease of the joints that develops when uric acid crystals are deposited in the joints.**

1. Furosemide (Lasix) is a diuretic and has no impact on uric acid formation.
3. Prochlorperazine (Compazine) is an antiemetic and has no impact on uric acid formation.
4. Potassium chloride (K-Dur) is an electrolyte and has no impact on uric acid formation.

Pregnancy Category: C
Client Need: Physiological Integrity

1 5 - 6

③ **The nurse will anticipate the administration of naloxone (Narcan) for clients with heroin overdose. Naloxone is an opiate antagonist that is administered to clients who have taken an overdose of opiate (usually heroin). Narcan reverses respiratory and central nervous system depression.**

1. Triazolam (Halcion) is a sedative-hypnotic administered for the treatment of insomnia.
2. Diazepam (Valium) is administered to treat anxiety, seizures, and muscle cramps.
4. Haloperidol (Haldol) is an antipsychotic; its use includes the treatment of psychotic symptoms seen with cocaine abuse.

Pregnancy Category: B
Client Need: Physiological Integrity

1 5 - 7

④ **You will anticipate a prescription for flumazenil (Romazicon). Such a marked drop in the respiratory rate is most likely due to the effects of diazepam (Valium). Flumazenil (Romazicon) is an antidote for benzodiazepine (Valium) and affects the receptor sites of benzodiazepines, making it an effective antagonist.**

1. Fentanyl (Sublimaze) would be contraindicated. It is an opioid analgesic (agonist) whose side effects include respiratory depression.
2. Fluorouracil (Adrucil) is an antineoplastic agent that has no impact on respiratory depression.
3. Fluconazole (Diflucan) is an antifungal agent that has no impact on respiratory depression.

Pregnancy Category: C
Client Need: Physiological Integrity

1 5 - 8

① **Diphenhydramine (Benadryl) is an effective treatment for clients with urticaria. Urticaria is a disorder of the skin that usually appears as a result of an allergic reaction. It is manifested by raised red areas on the skin. Diphenhydramine (Benadryl) is an antihistamine whose inhibition of histamine action helps alleviate allergic reaction.**

2. Sulconazole nitrate (Exelderm) is an antifungal agent and has no impact on urticaria.
3. Terconazole (Terazol) is a vaginal antifungal and has no impact on urticaria.
4. Tetracycline hydrochloride (Topicycline) is an antiacne cream and has no impact on urticaria.

Pregnancy Category: B
Client Need: Physiological Integrity

1 5 - 9

③ **Probenecid (Benemid) is an antigout (uricosuric) that reduces serum uric acid crystals by inhibiting renal tubular reabsorption of uric acid. The uric acid crystals are then excreted in the urine.**

1. Colchicine interferes with the functions of white blood cells and prevents the inflammatory response to the presence of uric acid crystals.
2. Metolazone (Zaroxolyn) is a diuretic, diazide-like antihypertensive, whose side effects may cause an increase in uric acid and thereby promote gout attacks.
4. Allopurinol (Zyloprim) is an antigout agent (xanthene oxidase inhibitor) that lowers serum uric acid levels by interfering with uric acid production.

Pregnancy Category: B
Client Need: Safe, Effective Care Environment

15-10

(1) **To prevent the disulfiram-alcohol reaction (acetaldehyde syndrome) from occurring, clients should not be given disulfiram (Antabuse) for a minimum of 12 hours after their last intake of alcohol. Disulfiram (Antabuse) is administered to manage alcohol dependence. Symptoms of the disulfiram-alcohol reaction include: Nausea, vomiting, hypertension, profuse sweating, palpitations, flushing, chest pain, and dyspnea.**

2, 3, and 4. Antabuse may be administered no sooner than 12 hours after the last ingestion of alcohol.

Pregnancy Category: C

Client Need: Physiological Integrity

15-11

(4) **Strong acids, alkalis, corrosives, or petroleum distillates are poisons that should not be removed by inducing vomiting because they will cause additional damage to tissue during vomiting. Ipecac is an emetic (an agent that produces vomiting) used to promote vomiting in the early treatment of overdose and poisoning by noncaustic substances in the conscious client.**

1, 2, and 3. Overdose or poisoning with acetaminophen, gentamicin, and multivitamins may be treated with ipecac.

Pregnancy Category: C

Client Need: Safe, Effective Care Environment

15-12

(2) **You will anticipate a prescription for protamine sulfate. Protamine sulfate is a heparin antagonist (antidote) that neutralizes the anticoagulant effect of heparin. The effect of protamine sulfate is monitored by activated partial thromboplastin time (APTT). An APTT greater than 100 seconds signifies spontaneous bleeding.**

1. Promethazine hydrochloride is an antiemetic antihistamine agent and has no impact on blood coagulation.
3. Procainamide is an antiarrhythmic and has no impact on blood coagulation.
4. Propranolol is a beta-adrenergic blocking agent and has no impact on blood coagulation.

Pregnancy Category: C

Client Need: Physiological Integrity

15-13

① Epistaxis, bruising, and petechiae are adverse reactions to antigout therapy. Because colchicine and allopurinol (antigout medications) may cause thrombocytopenia (low platelet count), clients may experience prolonged clotting times and subsequent bleeding. Signs of bleeding may include epistaxis (nosebleed), bruising, and petechiae (small hemorrhagic spots on the skin).

2. Constipation and neuropathic leg are generally caused by use of opioids. Demerol (an opioid) is used for pain relief in gout.

3. Tinnitus and blurred vision are generally caused by other nonsteroidal anti-inflammatory drugs (NSAIDs) such as aspirin.

4. Warmth and feelings of flush are associated with vasodilators.

Pregnancy Category: Colchicine, C; Allopurinol, C

Client Need: Physiological Integrity

15-14

③ Painful contractions and increased uterine activity are expected benefits of oxytocin (Pitocin). Pitocin is administered to facilitate uterine contractions. Postpartum Pitocin is given to control bleeding and promote milk letdown.

1. The infusion should be stopped and the physician notified for contractions occurring more frequently than every 2 minutes.

2. The infusion should be stopped and the physician notified for contractions lasting 60 to 90 seconds or longer.

4. The infusion should be stopped and the physician notified for significant changes in fetal heart rate or indications of water intoxication in the mother (drowsiness, confusion, headache, anuria, hyponatremia, or hypochloremia).

Pregnancy Category: NR

Client Need: Physiological Integrity

15-15

① Radioactive iodine, which is used to treat hyperthyroidism, may not be used at any stage of pregnancy because this medication may pass through the placenta and destroy the baby's thyroid gland.

2 and 4. Radioactive iodine treatment is indicated for persons over 18 years of age with hyperthyroidism and toxic multinodular goiter.

3. Radioactive iodine can be used for elderly clients.

Pregnancy Category: Not to be used during pregnancy

Client Need: Health Promotion/Maintenance

1 5 - 1 6

④ **Fine-toothed combs (nit combs) are used to remove any nits on hair shafts. Lindane (Kwell) is used in the treatment of pediculosis (head lice) and scabies (itch mite). When applied to treat head lice, the shampoo kills live lice. However, the nits (the eggs of the lice) may continue to cling to the hair shafts.**

1. Kwell shampoo is applied once to treat head lice. It may be repeated in a week if needed.

2. All family members should be treated with Kwell shampoo because pediculosis (head lice) is highly contagious.

3. Kwell shampoo is a pediculicide (kills lice). It is not indicated in the treatment of eczema, dermatitis, or other skin conditions such as dandruff.

Pregnancy Category: B
Client Need: Physiological Integrity

1 5 - 1 7

④ **Allopurinol (Zyloprim) is indicated in the treatment of hyperuricemic gout attacks. Because this medication inhibits the production of uric acid, the uric acid level drops and hyperuricemic gout abates (subsides).**

1. Penicillin G potassium (Pfizerpen) is a penicillin antibiotic and has no impact on uric acid levels.

2 and 3. Aspirin (acetylsalicylic acid) and acetaminophen (Tylenol) are antipyretic analgesics that may provide temporary pain relief but will have no impact on uric acid levels.

Pregnancy Category: C
Client Need: Physiological Integrity

Common Abbreviations

ā	before		OD	right eye
ac	before meals		OS	left eye
AD	right ear		os	mouth
ad lib	as needed		oz	ounce
amp	ampule		p̄	after
AS	left ear		po	by mouth
AU	each ear		PR	rectally
bid	twice a day		prn	when needed
cap	capsule		PV	vaginally
cc	cubic centimeter; 1 cc = 1 ml		q	every
D/C	discontinue		qd	every day
dl	deciliter		qh	every hour
dr	dram		qid	four times a day
elix	elixir		qod	every other day
gm	gram		s̄	without
gr	grain		SA	sustained action
h	hour		SC	subcutaneous
hs	hour of sleep		SL	sublingual
IM	intramuscular		Sol	solution
IV	intravenous		SR	sustained release
kg	kilogram		ss	one half
KVO	keep vein open		stat	immediately
L	left		tab	tablet
l	liter		tbs	tablespoon
mg	milligram		tid	three times a day
mEq	milliequivalent		tinct	tincture
ml	milliliter		TPR	total parenteral nutrition
NG	nasogastric		tsp	teaspoon
NPO	nothing by mouth			

Drug Names and Pronunciations, Trade Names, and Classification(s)

{Drug names in parentheses are available in Canada only.}

Acetaminophen [a-seat-a-**mee**-noe-fen]
{Abenol}, Aceta, Actamin, Aminofen, Anacin-3, Apacet, APAP, {Apo-Acetaminophen}, Arthritis Pain Formula Aspirin-Free, Atasol, Banesin, Dapa, Datril, Dolanex, Dorcol Children's Fever and Pain Reducer, {Exdor}, Feverall, Genapap, Genebs, Helenol, Liquiprin, Meda Cap, Myapap, Neopap, Oraphen, Panadol, Panex, Paracetamol, Phenaphen, Redutemp, Ridenol, {Robigesic}, {Rounox}, Snaplets-FR, St. Joseph's Aspirin-Free, Suppap, Tapanol, Tempra, Tenol, Tylenol, Ty-Pap, Ty-Tap, Valadol, Valorin
Classifications:
Nonopioid analgesic, antipyretic

Acetylysteine [a-se-til-**sis**-teen]
Mucomyst, Mucosil
Classification:
Antidote to acetaminophen

Acyclovir [ay-**sye**-kloe-veer]
Zovirax
Classification:
Antiviral

Adenosine [a-**den**-oh-seen]
Adenocard
Classification:
Antiarrhythmic

Albumin [al-**bu**-min]
Classification:
Blood derivative

Albuterol [al-**byoo**-ter-ole]
{Novosalmol}, Proventil, salbutamol, Ventolin
Classification:
Bronchodilator (beta-adrenergic agonist)

Allopurinol [al-oh-**pure**-i-nole]
{Alloprin}, {Apo Allopurinol}, Lopurin, {Novo-purol}, {Purinol}, Zyloprim
Classification:
Antigout agent (xanthene oxidase inhibitor)

Alprazolam [al-**pra**-soe-lam]
{Apo-Alpraz}, {Novo-Alprazol}, {Nu-Alpraz}, Xanax
Classification:
Sedative/hypnotic (benzodiazepine)

Alteplase [**al**-te-plase]
Activase, {Activase rt-PA}, tissue plasminogen activator, t-PA
Classification:
Thrombolytic

Aluminum Hydroxide [a-**loo**-me-num]
AlternaGEL, Alucap, {Alugel}, Aluminet, Alu-tab, Amphojel, Basalgel, Dialume, Nephrox
Classifications:
Antacid, electrolyte modifier (hypophosphatemic)

Aminophylline [am-in-**off**-i-lin]
{Corophyllin}, {Palaron}, Phyllocontin, Truphylline
Classification:
Bronchodilator (phosphodiesterase inhibitor)

Amlodipine besylate [am-**loe**-di-peen] [**bye**-sye-late]
Norvasc
Classifications:
Antihypertensive (calcium channel blocker), antianginal

Amphotericin B [am-foe-**ter**-i-sin]
Fungizone
Classification:
Antifungal

Antihemophilic Factor [an-tee-hee-mee-**fill**-ik]
AHF-M, Factor VIII S.D., Hemofil M, Humate P,
Koate HP, Kogenate, Monoclate P, Profilate OSD,
Recombinate
Classifications:
Hemostatic, blood derivative

Aspirin [**as**-pir-in]
acetylsalicylic acid, {Apo-ASA}, {Apo-Asen},
{Arthrinol}, {Arthrisin}, {Artria S.R}, Aspirgum,
ASA, {Astrin}, Bayer Aspirin, Bayer Timed-
Release Arthritic Pain Formula {Coryphen},
Easprin, Ecotrin, 8-hour Bayer Timed Release,
Empirin, {Entrophen}, Genprin, Halfprin,
{Headstart}, Measurin, Norwich Aspirin,
{Riphen}, {Sal-Adult}, {Sal-Infant}, St. Joseph
Adult Chewable Aspirin, Therapy Bayer,
ZORprin
Classifications:
Nonopioid analgesic, nonsteroidal anti-inflamma-
tory, antipyretic, antiplatelet agent

Atenolol [a-**ten**-oh-lole]
{Apo-Atenolol}, Tenormin
Classifications:
Antihypertensive, beta-adrenergic blocker (selec-
tive), antianginal

Atropine [**a**-troe-peen)
Atropair, Atro-Pen, Atropisol, Isopto-Atropine,
I-Tropine, {Minims Atropine}, Ocu-Tropine
Classifications:
Anticholingeric (antimuscarinic), antiarrhythmic,
ophthalmic (mydriatic)

Beclomethasone [be-kloe-**meth**-a-sone]
Beclovent, Beconase, Beconase AQ Nasal,
Vancenase, Vancenase AQ Nasal, Vanceril
Classification:
Glucocorticoid (long-acting)

Betamethasone Valerate [bay-ta-**meth**-a-sone]
Alphatrex, Betatrex, Valisone, Valnac
Classification:
Corticosteroid

Bethanechol chloride [be-**than**-e-kole]
DuVoid, Myotonochol, Urebeth, Urechloine,
Urolax
Classification:
Cholinergic (direct-acting)

Bisacodyl [bis-a-**koe**-dill]
{Bisacolax}, Bisco-Lax, Carter's Little Pills,
Dacodyl, Deficol, Dulcogen, Dulcolax, Fleet
Laxative, {Laxit}, Theralax
Classification:
Laxative (stimulant)

Botulinum [bot-u-**lee**-num]
Classification:
Antitoxin

Bromocriptine [broe-moe-**krip**-teen]
Parlodel
Classification:
Antiparkinsonian

Bumetanide [byoo-**met**-a-nide]
Bumex
Classification:
Diuretic (loop)

Calcitonin [kal-si-**toe**-nin]
Salmon: Calcimar, Miacalcin. Human: Cibacalcin
Classifications:
Hormone, electrolyte modifier (hypocalcemic)

Calcium carbonate [**kal**-see-um] [**kar**-boh-nate]
Cal Carb-Hd, Calciday, Cal-Sup, Caltrate,
Gencalc, Nephro-calci, Os-Cal, Oysco, Oystcal,
Titrilac, Tums
Classification:
Electrolyte

Carbamazepine [kar-ba-**maz**-e-peen]
{Apo-Carbamazepine}, Epitol, {Mazepine}, {Novo Carbamaz}, Tegretol
Classification:
Anticonvulsant

Carbamide peroxide [**kar**-ba-mid]
Murine Ear
Classification:
Otic

Carbidopa-Levodopa [**kar**-bi-doe-pa] [**lee**-voe-doe-pa]
Sinemet, Sinemet CR
Classification:
Antiparkinsonian

Cefazolin [sef-**a**-zoe-lin]
Ancef, Kefzol, Zolicef
Classification:
Anti-infective (cephalosporin)

Cefoxitin [se-**fox**-i-tin]
Mefoxin
Classification:
Anti-infective (second-generation cephalosporin)

Ceftriaxone [cef-try-**ax**-one]
Rocephin
Classification:
Anti-infective (third-generation cephalosporin)

Chloramphenicol [klor-am-**fen**-i-kole]
AK-Chlor, Chlorofair, Chloromycetin, Chloroptic, Econochlor, {Fenicol}, {Novochlorocap}, Ocu-Chlor, Ophthochlor, {Pentamycetin}, {Sopamycetin}, Spectro-Chlor
Classification:
Anti-infective

Chlordiazepoxide hydrochloride [klor-dye-az-e-**pox**-ide]
Librium
Classification:
Antianxiety agent

Chlortetracycline [klor-te-tra-**sye**-kleen]
Aureomycin Ointment 3%, Aureomycin Ophthalmic 1%
Classification:
Anti-infective (tetracycline)

Cholestyramine [koe-less-**tear**-a-meen]
Cholybar, Questran, Questran Light
Classification:
Lipid-lowering agent

Cimetidine [sye-**met**-i-deen]
{Apo-Cimetidine}, {Novocimetine}, {Peptol}, Tagamet
Classification:
Antiulcer (histamine H_2 antagonist)

Clofibrate [kloe-**fye**-brate]
Atromid-S, Claripex, Novofibrate
Classification:
Cholesterol-lowering agent

Clotrimazole [kloe-**try**-my-zole]
{Canesten}, Gyne-Lotrimin, Lotrimin, Mycelex-7, Mycelex-G, Mycelex-OTC
Classification:
Anti-infective

Colchicine [**kol**-chi-seen]
Classification:
Antigout agent

Colestipol [koe-less-**tip**-ole]
Colestid
Classification:
Lipid-lowering agent

Cromolyn sodium [**kro**-my-lon]
Crolom, Gastrocrom, Intal Spray Aerosol, Nasalcrom
Classification:
Miscellaneous respiratory agent

Cyanocobalamin [sye-an-oh-koe-**bal**-a-min]
Anacobin, Bedoz, Berubigen, Betalin 12, Cobex, Crystamine, Crysti-12, Cyanabin, Cyanoject, Kayborite, Redisol, Rubesol, Rubion, Rubramin PC, Sytobex, Vitamin B_{12}
Classification:
Vitamin B_{12}

Cyclobenzaprine [sye-kloe-**ben**-za-preen]
Cycloflex, Flexeril
Classification:
Skeletal muscle relaxant (centrally acting)

Cyclosporine [**sye**-kloe-spor-een]
Ciclosporin, Cyclosporin A, Sandimmune
Classification:
Immunosuppressant

Desoximetasone [des-ox-i-**met**-a-sone]
Topicort
Classifications:
Anti-inflammatory, topical glucocorticoid

Dexamethasone [dex-a-**meth**-a-sone]
Aeroseb-Dex, Decaderm, Decadron, Decaspray, Deronil, Dexameth, Dexamethasone Intensol, Dexasone, Dexone, Hexadrol, Maxidex, Mymethasone
Classifications:
Anti-inflammatory, glucocorticoid, antiemetic, corticosteroid, diagnostic

Dextroamphetamine [dex-troe-am-**fet**-a-meen]
Dexedrine, Ferndex, Oxydess II, Spancap #1
Classification:
CNS stimulant

Diazepam [dye-**az**-e-pam]
{Apo-Diazepam}, {Diazemuls}, {Novodipam}, T-Quil, Valium, Valrelease, Vazepam, {Vivol}, Zetran
Classifications:
Sedative/hypnotic (benzodiazepine), anticonvulsant (benzodiazepine), skeletal muscle relaxant (centrally acting)

Diazoxide [dye-az-**ox**-ide]
Hyperstat, Proglycem
Classifications:
Antihypertensive (vasodilator), hyperglycemic

Digitoxin [di-ji-**tox**-in]
Crystodigin
Classifications:
Cardiac glycoside, inotropic agent, antiarrhythmic

Digoxin [di-**jox**-in]
Lanoxicaps, Lanoxin, {Novodigoxin}
Classifications:
Cardiac glycoside, inotropic agent, antiarrhythmic

Diltiazem [dil-**tye**-a-zeem]
{Apo-Diltiaz}, Cardizem, Cardizem SR, Cardizem DC, Dilacor XR
Classifications:
Calcium channel blocker, antianginal, coronary vasodilator

Diphenhydramine [dye-fen-**hye**-dra-meen]
{Allerdryl}, AllerMax, Belix, Bena-D, Benadryl, Benahist, Ben-Allergin, Benaphen, Benoject, Benylin, Bydramine, Dihydrex, Diphen, Diphenacen, Diphenadryl, Dormarex 2, Genahist, Gen-D-phen, Hydramine, Hydramyn, Hyrexin, {Insomnal}, Maximum Strength Nytol, Nervine Nighttime Sleep-Aid, Nidryl, Nordryl, Phendry, Sleep-Eze 3, Sominex, Tusstat, Twilite, Valdrene, Wehdryl
Classifications:
Antihistamine, antitussive

Diphenoxylate hydrochloride/atropine [dye-fen-**ox**-i-late]
Diphenatol, Lofene, Logen, Lomanate, Lomotil, Lonox, Lo-Trol, Normil
Classification:
Antidiarrheal

Disopyramide [dye-soe-**peer**-a-mide]
Norpace, Norpace CR, {Rythmodan},
{Raythmodan-LA}
Classification:
Antiarrhythmic (group I)

Disulfiram [dye-**sul**-fi-ram]
Antabuse
Classification:
Alcohol abuse deterrent

Divalproex Sodium [dye-val-**pro**-ex] [**soe**-dee-um]
Depakote, {Epival}
Classification:
Anticonvulsant

Docusate sodium [**dok**-yoo-sate]
Colace, Dioeze, Diocto, Diosul, Disonate, DOK,
DOS Softgels, DOSS, Doxinate, DSS, Laxinate
100, Modane Soft, Regulax SS, {Regulex}, Regutol,
Therevac, Therevac SB
Classification:
Laxative (stool softener)

Dopamine [**doe**-pa-meen]
Dopastat, Intropin, {Revimine}
Classifications:
Vasopressor, inotropic agent

Dornase alfa [**dor**-nas]
Pulmozyme
Classification:
Miscellaneous respiratory agent

Doxorubicin [dox-oh-**roo**-bi-sin]
Adriamycin PFS, Adriamycin RDF, Rubex
Classification:
Antineoplastic (anthracycline)

Edrophonium [ed-roe-**fone**-ee-yum]
Enon, Reversol, Tensilon
Classification:
Cholinergic (anticholinesterase)

Enalapril [e-**nal**-a-pril]
Vasotec

Classifications:
Antihypertensive, angiotensin-converting
enzyme (ACE) inhibitor

Epinephrine (parenteral) [ep-i-**nef**-rin]
Adrenalin, AsthmaHaler, Bronkaid, Dysne-Inhal,
Medihaler-Epi, Primatene
Classifications:
Bronchodilator (adrenergic), cardiac stimulant,
ophthalmic (antiglaucomal)

Erythromycin [er-ith-roe-**mye**-sin]
Base: {Apo-Erythro-EC}, E-Base, E-Mycin,
{Erybid}, Eryc, Eryc-Sprinkle, Ery-tab,
{Erythromid}, PCE Dispersatabs, Robimycin.
Estolate: Erythrozone, Ilosone, {Novorythro}.
Ethyl-Succinate: {Apo-Erythro-ES}, E.E.S,
EryPed, Erythro. **Lactobionate:** Erythrocin.
Stearate: Eramycin, Erythrocin, {Novorythro},
Erythrocot, My-E, Wintrocin, Wyamycin S.
Ophthalmic: Ilotycin. **Topical:** Akne-Mycin,
Erycette, Erygel, Erymax, ETS, Mythromycin,
Staticin, T-stat.
Classification:
Anti-infective (macrolide)

Ethinyl estradiol [**eth**-i-nil]
Estinyl
Classification:
Hormonal (estrogen)

Famciclovir [fam-**sys**-kloe-ver]
Famvir
Classification:
Antiviral

Famotidine [fa-**moe**-ti-deen]
Pepcid
Classifications:
Histamine H$_2$ receptor antagonist, antiulcer agent

Fentanyl (parenteral) [**fen**-ta-nil]
Sublimaze
Classification:
Opioid analgesic (agonist)

Fentanyl (transdermal) [fen-ta-nil]
Duragesic
Classification:
Opioid analgesic (agonist)

Ferrous sulfate [fer-us sul-fate]
{Apo-Ferrous Sulfate}, Feosol, Fer-In-Sol, Fer-Iron, {Fero-Grad}, Fero-Gradumet, Ferralyn, Ferra-TD, Mol-Iron, {Novoferrosulfa}, {PMS Ferrous Sulfate}, Slow Fe
Classifications:
Antianemic, iron supplement

Fluconazole [floo-kon-a-zole]
Diflucan
Classification:
Antifungal

Flucytosine [floo-sye-toe-seen]
Ancobon, {Ancotil}, 5-FC
Classification:
Antifungal

Fludarabine [floo-dar-a-been]
Fludara
Classification:
Antineoplastic (antimetabolite)

Flumazenil [flu-maz-e-nil]
Romazicon
Classification:
Antidote (benzodiazepine antagonist)

Fluorouracil [flure-oh-yoor-a-sil]
Adrucil, Efudex, Fluoroplex, 5-FU
Classification:
Antineoplastic (antimetabolite)

Fluoxetine [floo-ox-uh-teen]
Prozac
Classification:
Antidepressant

Folic acid [foe-lik as-id]
{Apo-Folic}, Folate, Folvite, {Novofolacid}, Vitamin B_9

Classifications:
Vitamin (water-soluble), antianemic

Furosemide [fur-oh-se-mide]
{Apo-Furosemide}, {Furoside}, Lasix, Myrosemide, {Novosemide}, {Uritol}
Classification:
Diuretic (loop)

Ganciclovir [gan-sys-kloe-vir]
Cytovene
Classification:
Antiviral

Gentamicin [jen-ta-mye-sin]
{Alcomicin}, {Cidomycin}, Garamycin, Genoptic, Gentafair, Gentak, Gentrasul, G-Mycon, Jenamicin, Ocu-Mycin, Spectro-Genta
Classification:
Anti-infective (aminoglycoside)

Glipizide [glip-i-zide]
Glucotrol
Classification:
Oral hypoglycemic agent (sulfonylureas)

Glucagon [gloo-ka-gon]
Classification:
Hormone (pancreatic)

Glyburide [gli-bu-ride]
Glynase, Glynase Pres Tab, Micronase
Classification:
Hormonal (antidiabetic)

Griseofulvin microsize [gris-ee-oh-ful-vin]
Grifulvin, Grisacton, Grisovin
Classification:
Local anti-infective

Haloperidol [ha-loe-per-i-dole]
{Apo-Haloperidol}, Haldol, Haldol Decanoate, {Haldo L.A.}, {Novoperidol}, {Peridol}
Classification:
Antipsychotic (butyrophenone)

Heparin sodium [**hep**-a-rin]
{Calcilean}, Calciparine, {Hepalean}, {Heparin Leo}, Liquaemin
Classification:
Anticoagulant

Hetastarch [**het**-a-starch]
Hespan
Classification:
Volume expander

Hydrochlorothiazide [hye-droe-klor-oh-**thye**-a-zide] {Apo-Hydro}, {Duiclor H}, Esidrex, Ezide, HCTZ, HydroDIURIL, Hydro-Par, {Natrimax}, {Neo-Codema}, Novo-Hydrazide, Oretic, {Urozide}
Classifications:
Diuretic (thiazide), antihypertensive

Ibuprofen [eye-byoo-**proe**-fen]
Aches-N-Pain, {Acitprofen}, Advil, {Amersol}, {Apo-Ibuprofen}, Children's Motrin, Excedrin IB, Genpril, Haltran, Ibuprin, Ibuprohm, Ibu-Tab, Medipren, Midol 200, Notrin, Motrin IB, {Novoprofen}, Nurpin, Pamprin-IB, Rufen, Saleto, Trendar
Classifications:
Nonsteroidal anti-inflammatory agent, nonopioid analgesic, antipyretic

Idoquinol [eye-oh-do-**kwin**-ole]
Diiodohydroxyquin, Diodoquin, Moebiquin, Sebaquin, Yodoxin
Classifications:
Anti-infective, antiprotozoal, amebicide

Indomethacin [in-doe-**meth**-a-sin]
Indocin, Indocin-SR
Classification:
Nonsteroidal anti-inflammatory

Insulin [**in**-su-lin]
Rapid-acting: Regular (Actrapid, Humulin R, Iletin I, Iletin II, Iletin II U-500 [concentrated], Novolin R, Velosulin); prompt zinc suspension (Semilente, Semilente Iletin, Semitard)

Intermediate-acting: isophane suspension (Humulin N, Iletin II, Insultard NPH, Lentard, Novolin N, NPH, NPH Purified); zinc suspension (Humulin L, Lente, Lente Iletin, Monotard, Novolin L)

Long-acting: extended zinc suspension (Humulin U, Ultralente, Ultralente Iletin, Ultratard)

Insulin Mixture: Regular plus NPH (Humulin 70/30, Mixtard 70/30, Novolin 70/30)
Classification:
Hormone (pancreatic)

Interferon Alfa-2b [in-ter-**feer**-on]
a-2-interferon, Intron A
Classifications:
Antineoplastic, antiviral, immunomodulator

Ipecac Syrup [**ip**-e-kak]
Classification:
Emetic

Iron Dextran [**eye**-ern **dex**-tran]
{Imferon}, InFeD
Classifications:
Antianemic, iron supplement

Ketorolac [kee-**toe**-role-ak]
Toradol
Classifications:
Nonopioid analgesic, nonsteroidal anti-inflammatory

Leucovorin [loo-koe-**vor**-in]
Citrovorum factor, 5-Formyl Tetrahydrofolate, Folinic Acid, Wellcovorin
Classifications:
Antidote (for methotrexate and folic acid antagonists), vitamin (folic acid analog)

Levamisole [lee-**vam**-i-sole]
Ergamisole
Classification:
Antineoplastic (immunomodulator)

Levodopa [**lee**-voe-doe-pa]
Dopar, Larodopa, L-Dopa
Classification:
Antiparkinsonian (dopamine agonist)

Levothyroxine [lee-voe-thye-**rox**-een]
{Eltroxin}, Levothroid, Levoxine, Synthroid, T_4
Classification:
Hormone (thyroid)

Lidocaine [**lye**-doe-kane]
Anestacon, Baylocaine, L-Caine, LidoPen,
Xylocaine, {Xylogard}
Classifications:
Antiarrhythmic (group IB), anesthetic (local)

Lindane [**lin**-dane]
Bio-well, Gamma benzene hexachloride, GBH,
G-well, Kwell, {Kwellada}, Kwildane, Scabene,
Thionex
Classification:
Antiparasitic

Mafenide acetate [**maf**-en-id]
Sulfamylon
Classification:
Local anti-infective

Mannitol [**man**-i-tol]
Osmitrol
Classification:
Diuretic (osmotic)

Mebendazole [me-**ben**-da-zole]
{Nemasole}, Vermox
Classification:
Antihelmintic

Meperidine Hydrochloride [me-**per**-I-deen]
[hy-droe-**klor**-ide]
Demerol, Pethadol, Pethidine
Classification:
Opioid analgesic (agonist)

Methocarbamol [meth-oh-**kar**-ba-mole]
Delaxin, Marbaxin, Robaxin, Robomol

Classification:
Skeletal muscle relaxant (centrally acting)

Methotrexate [meth-o-**trex**-ate]
Amethopterin, Folex, Folex PFS, Rheumatrex
Classifications:
Antineoplastic (antimetabolite),
immunosuppressant

Metolazone [me-**tole**-a-zone]
Mykrox, Zarozolyn
Classifications:
Diuretic (thiazide-like), antihypertensive

Metoprolol [me-**toe**-proe-lole]
{Apo-Metoprolol}, {Betaloc}, {Betaloc Durules},
Lopressor, {Lopressor SR}, {Novometoprol},
Toprop XL
Classifications:
Antihypertensive, antianginal, beta-adrenergic
blocker (selective)

Metronidazole [me-troe-**ni**-da-zole]
{Apo-Metronidazole}, Flagyl, Metizol, Metric 21,
MetroGel, Metro IV, Metryl, Metryl IV, {Neo-
Metric}, {Novonidazoel}, {PMS Metrodiazole},
Protostat, Satric, {Trikacide}
Classification:
Anti-infective

Morphine sulfate [**mor**-feen]
Astramorph PF, Duramorph, {Epimorph},
{Morphine H.P.}, {Morphitec}, {M.O.S.}, M.O.S.-
S.R.}, MS, MSO_4, MS Contin, MSIR, MSIR
Capsules, OMS Concentrate, Oramorph SR, RMS,
Roxanol, Roxanol SR {Statex}
Classification:
Opioid analgesic (agonist)

Nalbuphine [**nal**-byoo-feen]
Nubain
Classification:
Opioid analgesic (agonist/antagonist)

Naloxone [nal-**ox**-one]
Narcan

Classification:
Antidote (for opioids}

Naproxen sodium [na-**prox**-en]
Aleve, Anaprox, Anaprox DS, Naprelan
Classification:
Nonsteroidal anti-inflammatory

Neomycin [nee-oh-**mye**-sin]
Mycifradin, Myciguent
Classification:
Anti-infective (aminoglycoside)

Nifedipine [nye-**fed**-i-peen]
Adalat, Adalat CC, {Adalat P.A.}, {Apo-Nifed},
{Novo-Nifedin}, {NuNifed}, Procardia, Procardia
XL
Classifications:
Calcium channel blocker, antianginal, coronary
vasodilator, antihypertensive

Nitroglycerin [nye-troe-**gli**-ser-in]
Nitroglycerin extended-release capsules:
Nitrobid, Nitrocap T.D., Nitrocine, Nitroglyn,
Nitrolin; **Nitroglycerin extended-release tablets:**
Klavikordal, Niong, Nitronet, Nitrong; **Nitro-
glycerin extended-release buccal tablets:**
Nitrogard, {Nitrogard SR}; **Nitroglycerin intra-
venous:** Nitro-bid, Tridil; **Nitroglycerin lingual
spray:** Nitrolingual; **Nitroglycerin ointment:**
Nitro-bid, Nitrol, Nitrong; **Nitroglycerin sublin-
gual:** Nitrostat; **Nitroglycerin transdermal:**
Deponit, Minitran, Nitrodisc, Nitro-Dur, Nitro-
Dur II, NTS, Transderm-Nitro
Classifications:
Vasodilator (nitrate), antianginal, coronary
vasodilator

Nitroprusside [nye-troe-**pruss**-ide]
Nitropress
Classification:
Antihypertensive (vasodilator)

Nizatidine [ni-**za**-ti-deen]
Axid
Classifications:
Histamine H_2 antagonist, antiulcer

Norepinephrine [**nor**-ep-i-nef-rin]
Levarterenol, Levophed
Classification:
Vasopressor

Nortriptyline Hydrochloride [nor-**trip**-ti-leen]
[hy-droe-**klor**-ide]
Aventyl, Pamelor
Classification:
Antidepressant (tricyclic)

Nystatin [nye-**stat**-in]
Mycostatin, {Nadostine}, {Nyaderm}, Nystex
Classification:
Antifungal

Oxamniquine [ox-**am**-ni-kwin]
Vansil
Classification:
Anthelmintic

Oxytocin [ox-i-**toe**-sin]
Pitocin, Syntocinon
Classification:
Hormone (oxytocic)

Paclitaxel [pa-kli-**tax**-el]
Taxol
Classification:
Antineoplastic (antimicrotubule agent)

Pancrelipase [pan-kree-**li**-pase]
Catozym, Cotazym-S, Cotazym-65 B, Cotazym
E.C.S. 8, Cotazym E.C.S. 20, Enzymase-16,
Ilozyme, Ku-Zume HP, Pancrease, Pancrease
MT 4, Pancrease MT 10, Pancoate, Pancrease
MT 16, Protilase, Ultrase MT 12, Ultrase MT 20,
Ultrase MT 24, Viokase, Zymase
Classification:
Pancreatic

Paroxetine [par-**ox**-e-teen]
Paxil
Classification:
Antidepressant

Penicillin G Procaine [pen-i-**sill**-in] [jee] [**proe**-cane]
{Ayercillin}, Crysticillin A.S., Pfizerpen-AS, Wycillin
Classification:
Anti-infective (penicillin)

Pentaerythritol Tetranitrate [pen-ta-er-**ith**-ri-tole tet-ra-**nye**-trate]
Duotrate, Naptrate, Pentol, Pentritol, Pentylan, Peritrate, P.E.T.N.
Classifications:
Vasodilator, antianginal, nitrate

Pentamidine [pen-**tam**-i-deen]
Nebupent, Pentam, {Pentacarinat}, {Pneumopent}
Classification:
Anti-infective (antiprotozoal)

Phenytoin [**fen**-i-toyn]
Dyphenylhydantoin, DPH, Dilantin, Diphenylan
Classifications:
Anticonvulsant (hydantoin), antiarrhythmic (group IB)

Pilocarpine [pye-loe-**kar**-peen]
Adsorbocarpine, Akarpine, Isopto Carpine, Ocu-Carpine, Pilagan, Pilocar, Piloptic, Pilostat, Pilopto-Carpine, Ocusert-Pilo
Classification:
Ophthalmic cholinergic agent (direct-acting)

Piperazine Adipate [**pi**-per-a-zeen][**add**-i-pate]
{Entacyl}
Classification:
Anthelmintic

Potassium Chloride [poe-**tass**-ee-um]
Apo-K, Cena-K, Gen-K, K-10, {Kalium Durules}, Kaochlor, Kaochlor S-F, Kaon Cl, Kato, Kay Ciel, KCI, K-Dur, {K-Long}, K- Lor, Klor-10%, Klor-Con, Klorvess, Klotrix, K-Lyte / Cl Powder, K- Norm, K+Care, K+10, K-Lease, {K-Long], K-Tab, Micro-K, LS, {Novolente-K}, Potachlor, Potasalan, Rum-K, Slow-K, Ten-K
Classification:
Electrolyte (potassium supplement)

Prazosin [pra-**zoe**-in]
Minipress
Classification:
Antihypertensive (peripherally acting anti-adrenergic)

Prednisolone [pred-**niss**-oh-lone]
Articulose, Delta-Cortef, Hydeltra-T.B.A., Hyudeltrasol, Key-Pred, Nor-Pred T.B.A., Pediapred, Predaject, Predalone, Predalone T.B.A., Predate, Predocor, Predicort, Prednisol, Prelone
Classification:
Glucocorticoid (intermediate-acting)

Prednisone [**pred**-ni-sone]
{Apo-Prednisone}, Deltasone, Liquid Pred, Meticorten, Orasone, Panasol, Prednicen-M, Sterapred, {Winpred}
Classification:
Glucocorticoid (intermediate-acting)

Probenecid [proe-**ben**-e-sid]
Benemid, {Benuryl}, Probalan
Classification:
Antigout agent (uricosuric)

Procainamide [pro-**kane**-ah-mide]
Procan SR, Promine, Pronestyl, Pronestyl-SR
Classification:
Antiarrhythmic (group IA)

Prochlorperazine [proe-klor-**pair**-a-zeen]
Chlorpazine, Compa-Z, Compazine, Contranzine, {Provazin}, {Stemetil}, Ultrazine
Classifications:
Antiemetic (phenothiazine), antipsychotic

Promethazine [**proe**-meth-a-zeen]
Anergan, {Histanil}, Mallergan, Pentazine, Phenameth, Phenazine, Phencen-50, Phenergan, Phenergan Fortis, Phenergan Plain, Phenoject-50, {PMS Promethazine}, Pro-50, Prometh-25, Prometh-50, Prorex, Prothazine Plain, Remsed, V-Gan
Classifications:
Antihistamine (phenothiazine), antiemetic, sedative / hypnotic

Propranolol [proe-**pran**-oh-lole]
{Apo-Propranolol}, {Detensol}, Inderal, Inderal-LA, {Novopranol}
Classifications:
Antihypertensive, antianginal, beta-adrenergic blocker (nonselective), antiarrhythmic

Protamine Sulfate [**proe**-ta-meen]
Classification:
Antidote (antiheparin agent)

Pseudoephedrine [soo-doe-e-**fed**-rin]
Afrin, Drixoral
Classification:
Adrenergic (sympathomimetic)

Pyridostigmine bromide [peer-id-oh-**stig**-meen]
Mestinon, Mestinon Timespan, Regonol
Classification:
Cholinergic (anticholinesterase)

Quinidine gluconate [**kwin**-i-deen]
Duraquin, Quinaglute, Quinlan
Classification:
Antiarrhythmic

Ramipril [**ram**-i-pril]
Altace
Classification:
Antihypertensive (angiotensin-converting enzyme (ACE) inhibitor

Ranitidine [ra-**nye**-te-deen]
{Apo-Ranitidine}, Zantac, {Zantac-C}
Classifications:
Histamine H_2 antagonist, antiulcer

Rh$_0$ (D) Immune Globulin [**arr**-aych-oh] {dee} [im-**yoon**] [**glob**-yoo-lin]
Standard dose: Gamulin Rh, HypRho-D, Rhesonativ, RhoGam; Microdose: HypRho-D Mini-Dose, MICRhoGam, Mini-Gamulin Rh
Classification:
Immune globulin

Ritodrine Hydrochloride [**ri**-toe-dreen] [hye-droe-**klor**-ide]
Yutopar
Classifications:
Beta-adrenergic agonist, tocolytic

Rubella virus vaccine [roo-**bel**-a]
Meruvax II
Classification:
Immunomodulator (vaccine)

Silver nitrate [**sil**-ver] [**nye**-trate]
Ophthalmic solution 1%
Classification:
Ophthalmic anti-infective

Silver Sulfadiazine [**sil**-ver] [sul-fa-**dye**-a-zeen]
{Flamazine}, Flint SSD, Silvadene, Thermazene
Classification:
Anti-infective (topical)

Sodium Bicarbonate [**soe**-dee-um] [bye-**kar**-boe-nate]
Baking Soda, Bellans, Citrocarbonate, Neut, Soda Mint
Classifications:
Electrolyte modifier (alkalinizing agent, antacid)

Sodium Polystyrene Sulfonate [**soe**-dee-um] [pa-lee-**stye**-reen] [sul-**fon**-ate]
Kayexalate, SPS
Classification:
Electrolyte modifier (cation exchange resin)

Spironolactone [speer-oh-no-**lak**-tone]
Aldactone, {Novospiroton}
Classification:
Diuretic (potassium-sparing)

Streptomycin [strep-toe-**mye**-sin]
Classifications:
Anti-infective (aminoglycoside), antitubercular

Sucralfate [soo-**kral**-fate]
Carafate, {Sulcrate}
Classification:
Antiulcer agent (protectant)

Sulconazole Nitrate [sul-**kon**-a-zole] [**nye**-trate]
Exelderm
Classification:
Antifungal (topical)

Sulfasalazine [sul-fa-**sal**-a-zen]
Azulfidine
Classification:
Miscellaneous uncategorized drug

Tamoxifen [ta-**mox**-i-fen]
Nolvadex, {Nolvades-D}, {Novo-Tamoxifen},
{Tamofen}, {Tamone}
Classification:
Antineoplastic (estrogen blocker)

Terbutaline [ter-**byoo**-ta-leen]
Brethaire, Brethine, Bricanyl
Classification:
Bronchodilator (beta-adrenergic agonist)

Terconazole [ter-**kon**-a-zole]
Terazol
Classification:
Antifungal (vaginal)

Tetracycline [te-tra-**sye**-kleen]
Achromycin, Alatet, {Apo-Tetra}, Nor-tet,
{Novotetra}, {Nu-Tetra}, Panmycin, Robitet,
Sumycin, Teline, Tetracap, Tetracyn, Tetralan,
Topicycline
Classification:
Anti-infective (tetracycline)

Theophylline [thee-**off-**i-lin]
Accurbron, Aerolate, Aquaphyllin, Asmalix,
Bronkodyl, Elixomin, Elixophyllin, Lanophyllin,
Lixolin {Pulmophylline}, Slophyllin Syrup,
Synophylate, Theoclear, Theolair, Theon,
Theophyl, Theostat
Extended Release: Aerolate, Constant-T,
Elixophyllin SR, LaBID, Quibron-T/SR, Respid,
Slo-bid Gyrocaps, Slophyllin, Sustaire, T- Phyl,
Theo-24, Theobid Duracap, Theobid Jr, Duracap,
Theochron, Theoclear LA, Theoclear LA Cenules,
Theo-Dur, Theo-Dur Sprinkle, Theolair-SR,

Theophyl-SR, Theospan-SR, Theo-Sav, Theo-
Time, Theovent Long-Acting, Uniphyl
Classification:
Bronchodilator (phosphodiesterase inhibitor)

Thiabendazole [thye-a-**ben**-a-zole]
Mintezol
Classifications:
Anthelmintic, enzyme inhibitor

Tolbutamide [tole-**byoo**-ta-mide]
{Apo-Tolbutamide}, {Mobenol}, {Novobutamide},
Oramide, Orinase
Classification:
Oral hypoglycemic agent (sulfonylureas)

Torsemide [**tor**-see-mide]
Classification:
Loop diuretic

Tranylcypromine sulfate [tran-il-**si**-pro-men]
Parnate
Classification:
Antidepressant

Triazolam [trye-**az**-oh-lam]
{Apo-Triazo}, Halcion, {Novotriolam},
{Nu-Triazo}
Classification:
Sedative/hypnotic (benzodiazepine)

Trihexyphenidyl hydrochloride [tyre-hex-ee-**fen**-
i-dill]
Artane, Artane Sequels, Trihexane
Classification:
Antiparkinsonian

Trimethoprim [trye-**meth**-oh-prim]
Proloprim, Trimpex
Classification:
Anti-infective

Triprolidine hydrochloride [trye-**proe**-li-deen]
Actidil, Alleract, Myidl
Classification:
Antihistamine

Tuberculin purified protein derivative (PPD)
[too-**bur**-que-lin]
Aplisol, PPD-Stabilized Solution
Classification:
Diagnostic

Vasopressin [vas-o-**pres**-in]
Pitressin
Classification:
Hormonal (pituitary)

Vecuronium [ve-**kure**-oh-nee-yum]
Norcuron
Classification:
Neuromuscular blocking agent (nondepolarizing)

Verapamil [ver-**ap**-a-mil]
Calan, Calan SR, Isoptin, Isoptin SR, Verelan
Classifications:
Calcium channel blocker, antianginal, antihypertensive, antiarrhythmic, coronary vasodilator

Vincristine [vin-**kriss**-teen]
Oncovin, Vincasar PFS
Classification:
Antineoplastic agent (vinca alkaloid)

Vitamin A (beta carotene) [**vye**-ta-min A]
Aquasol A, Del-Vi-A
Classification:
Vitamin (fat-soluble)

Vitamin B (dexpanthenol) [dex-**pan**-the-nole]
Llopan, Panthoderm
Classifications:
Cholinergic (direct-acting); vitamin B complex

Vitamin B$_6$ (pyridoxine) [peer-i-**dox**-een]
Beesix, {Hexa-Betalin}, Nestrex, Rodex, Vitabee 6, Vitamin B$_6$
Classification:
Vitamin (water-soluble)

Vitamin C (ascorbic acid) [as-**kor**-bic-] [**as**-id]
Vitamin C, {Apo-C}, Ascorbicap, Cecon, Cemill, Cetane, Cevalin, Ce-Vi-Sol, Flavorcee
Classification:
Vitamin (water-soluble)

Vitamin D (dihydrotachysterol) [dye-hye-droe-tak-**iss**-ter-ole]
DNT, DHT Intensol, Hytakerol
Classifications:
Vitamin D, serum calcium regulator

Vitamin K$_1$ (phytonadione) [fye-toe-na-**dye**-one]
AquaMEPHYTON, Konakion, Mephyton
Classification:
Vitamin (fat-soluble)

Warfarin sodium [**war**-far-in]
Coumadin, Sofarin, {Warfilone}
Classification:
Anticoagulant

FDA Pregnancy Risk Categories

The developing fetus of a pregnant woman is at potential risk for birth defects and death when exposed to medications. The U.S. Food and Drug Administration (FDA) has authorized five categories (Categories A, B, C, D, and X) that indicate some medications' potential for producing birth defects or fetal death. The identifying letters signal the level of risk to the fetus. The risks follow a continuum from safe to unsafe. Medications in Category A are generally viewed as safe for pregnant women, whereas medications in Category X are generally deemed unsafe and are contraindicated.

Category	Description
A	Controlled studies in pregnant women have not demonstrated a risk to the fetus. The potential for fetal harm appears remote.
B	Somewhat more of a risk to the fetus than Category A. Animal studies show no risk to a fetus. However, studies have not been completed in women—or, animal studies do indicate a risk to the fetus, but studies in women do not indicate a risk.
C	Greater risk than Category B. Animal studies do show a risk of fetal harm. However, no studies have been completed in women—or no studies have been completed in women or animals.
D	Proven risk of harm to the fetus. Studies in pregnant women provide proof of fetal damage. This medication should be used only if the risk of the untreated condition for the woman is greater than the risk of the medication for the fetus. A statement of fetal risk will appear in the WARNING section of medication labeling.
X	Proven risk of harm to the fetus. Studies in pregnant women and animals indicate definite risk of fetal abnormalities. Fetal risks outweigh all possible benefits. A statement of risk appears in the CONTRAINDICATIONS section of medication labeling.

Table of Measurement Equivalents

Health-care providers prescribing, dispensing, and/or administering medications should abide by the protocols of the facility where they work. When dosage calculations are required, they should be checked by a pharmacist before administering.

The following charts express approximate liquid and dry weights and their equivalents and conversions, with metric measures as the standard and apothecary and household (British imperial) measures afterward.

LIQUID MEASUREMENTS

Metric	Approximate Apothecary Equivalents	Approximate Household Equivalents
1000 ml	32 fluid ounces (1 quart)	1 quart
500 ml	16 fluid ounces (1 pint)	1 pint
250 ml	8 fluid ounces	1 cup
30 ml	1 fluid ounce	2 tablespoons
15 ml	4 fluid drams	1 tablespoon
4 or 5 ml	1 fluid dram	1 teaspoon
1 ml	15 or 16 minims	1/4 teaspoon
0.06 ml	1 minim	1 drop

[1 milliliter (ml) is the approximate equivalent of 1 cubic centimeter (cc).]

APPROXIMATE SOLID EQUIVALENTS

Avoirdupois	Apothecary
1 grain (gr)	1 grain (gr)
15.4 gr	15 gr
1 ounce	480 gr
1 pound (lb)	1.33 lb
2.2 lb	2.7 lb

WEIGHTS

Metric	Apothecary
30 gm	1 ounce
15 gm	4 drams
4 gm	60 grains (1 dram)
1 gm	15 or 16 grains
300 mg	5 grains
60 mg	1 grain
30 mg	1/2 grain
10 mg	1/6 grain
6 mg	1/10 grain
1 mg	1/60 grain
0.6 mg	1/100 grain
0.5 mg	1/120 grain
0.4 mg	1/150 grain
0.3 mg	1/200 grain
0.2 mg	1/300 grain
0.1 mg	1/600 grain

Metric Conversions

1 kg	=	1000 gm
1 gm	=	1000 mg
1 mg	=	0.001 gm
1 mcg	=	0.001 mg

1 gram (gm)	=	1000 milligrams (mg)
1000 grams	=	1 kilogram (kg)
.001 milligram	=	1 microgram (mcg)
1 meter	=	100 centimeters (cm)
1 meter	=	1000 millimeters (mm)

Conversion Equivalents

Metric	Metric Equivalents	Apothecary
1 gram (g)	1000 milligrams	15 grains
0.6 gram	600 milligrams	10 grains
0.5 gram	500 milligrams	7.5 grains
0.3 gram	300 milligrams	5 grains
0.06 gram	60 milligrams	1 grain

VOLUME

Metric	Apothecary	Household
1 milliliter	15 minims (M)	15 drops (gtt)
5 milliliters	1 fluid dram (ℨ)	1 teaspoon (tsp)
15 milliliters	4 fluid drams	1 tablespoon (T)
30 milliliters	1 ounce (oz)	2 tablespoons
500 milliliters	1 pint (pt)	1 pint (pt)
1000 milliliters	1 quart (qt)	1 quart (qt)

Conversion Equivalents

Metric	Metric Equivalents	Apothecary
1 liter (l)	1000 milliliters (ml)	1 quart (qt)
1 deciliter (dl)	100 milliliters (ml)	3.2 fluid ounces (fl oz)
1 milliliter (ml)	1 cubic centimeter (cc)	15 minims (M)

APOTHECARIES' METRIC

15 grains	=	1000 mg	1/6 grain	=	10 mg
10 grains	=	600 mg	1/10 grain	=	6 mg
5 grains	=	300 mg	1/15 grain	=	4 mg
1 1/2 grains	=	100 mg	1/20 grain	=	3 mg
1 grain	=	60 mg	1/30 grain	=	2 mg
3/4 grain	=	45 mg	1/60 grain	=	1 mg
2/3 grain	=	40 mg	1/100 grain	=	0.6 mg
1/2 grain	=	30 mg	1/200 grain	=	0.3 mg
3/8 grain	=	25 mg	1/250 grain	=	0.25 mg
1/3 grain	=	20 mg	1/300 grain	=	0.2 mg
1/4 grain	=	15 mg	1/600 grain	=	0.1 mg
1/5 grain	=	12 mg	1/1000 grain	=	0.06 mg

HOUSEHOLD METRIC

20 drops	=	1 ml
1 teaspoon	=	5 ml
1 tablespoon	=	15 ml

WEIGHT CONVERSIONS

1 oz	=	30 gm
1 lb	=	453.6 gm
2.2 lb	=	1 kg

LENGTH

1 cm	=	0.39 inch
1 inch	=	2.54 cm

CENTIGRADE/ FAHRENHEIT CONVERSIONS

C	=	(F - 32) x 5/9
F	=	(C x 9/5) +32